LOUISA CRONIN

THE ULTIMATE BLOOD TYPE A'S

DIET COOKBOOK FOR BEGINNERS

MASTER YOUR A: EASY AND DELICIOUS RECIPES FOR BLOOD TYPE A NEGATIVE AND POSITIVE INDIVIDUALS.

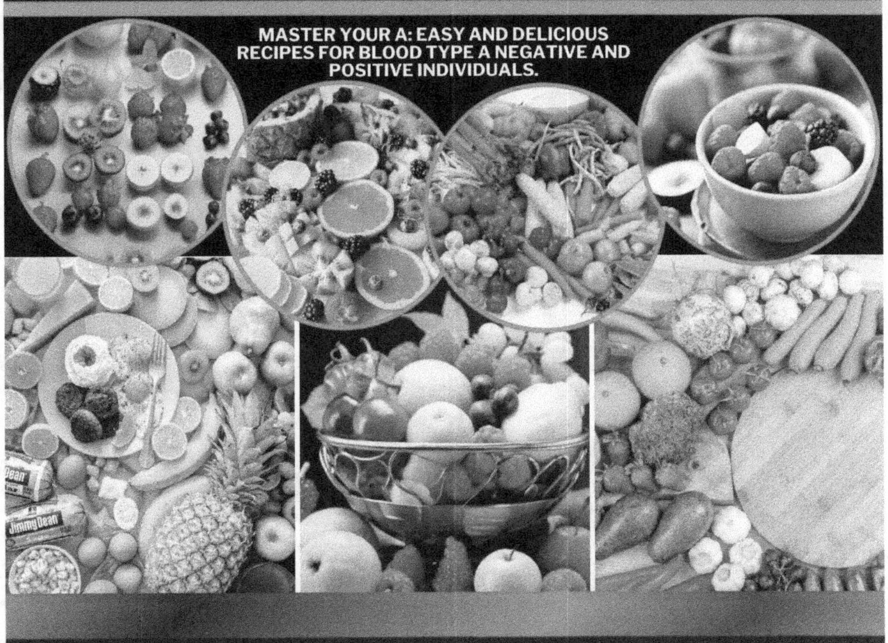

COPYRIGHT

TABLE OF CONTENTS

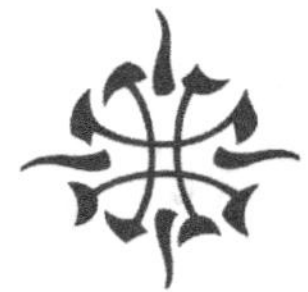

Introduction to Blood Type A Diets

The concept of blood type diets is based on the idea that individuals with different blood types should follow specific dietary guidelines to optimize their health and well-being. One popular version of this approach is the Blood Type A Diet, which is tailored for individuals with blood type A.

Understanding Blood Type A

People with blood type A are believed to have evolved from agricultural ancestors who relied heavily on plant-based diets. According to the blood type diet theory, individuals with blood type A have specific characteristics and sensitivities that make them more suitable for vegetarian or plant-based diets.

Benefits of Tailored Diets

Proponents of blood type diets claim that following a diet specific to your blood type can provide various benefits. Here are some potential benefits associated with the Blood Type A Diet:

1. Weight management: The Blood Type A Diet emphasizes plant-based foods, which are typically lower in calories and higher in fiber. This can help individuals with blood type A maintain a healthy weight or achieve weight loss goals.

2. Improved digestion: The diet recommends avoiding certain foods that are believed to be less compatible with blood type A. By avoiding these foods, individuals may experience improved digestion and reduced bloating or other digestive discomforts.

3. Enhanced immune function: The Blood Type A Diet encourages the consumption of whole, unprocessed foods, which are rich in essential nutrients and antioxidants. A nutrient-rich diet can support a healthy immune system, reducing the risk of infections and promoting overall well-being.

4. Reduced risk of chronic diseases: The diet's emphasis on plant-based foods, including fruits, vegetables, and whole grains, can provide a wide range of vitamins, minerals, and phytochemicals that are associated with a lower risk of chronic diseases, such as heart disease, diabetes, and certain types of cancer.

5. Increased energy levels: Proponents of the Blood Type A Diet suggest that following a diet aligned with your blood type can improve energy levels and reduce fatigue. This is attributed to the theory that certain foods may be more or less compatible with your blood type, affecting your body's ability to efficiently utilize nutrients for energy.

It's important to note that the scientific evidence supporting the blood type diet theory is limited and inconclusive. Many nutrition experts consider the blood type diets as lacking scientific basis and prefer a more individualized approach to dietary recommendations based on factors such as personal preferences, overall health, and specific nutritional needs.

Before making any significant changes to your diet, it's advisable to consult with a registered dietitian or healthcare professional who can provide personalized guidance based on your specific needs and health goals.

OVERVIEW OF BLOOD TYPE A DIETARY GUIDELINES

The Blood Type A Diet focuses on a predominantly vegetarian or plant-based approach. Here is an overview of the dietary guidelines for individuals with blood type A:

1. Emphasize plant-based foods: The foundation of the Blood Type A Diet is a variety of fruits, vegetables, legumes, whole grains, and plant-based proteins like tofu and tempeh. These foods are believed to be better suited for individuals with blood type A.

2. Limit animal products: The diet suggests reducing or eliminating animal products, particularly red meat and dairy, as they are considered less compatible with blood type A. However, small amounts of low-fat dairy products, fish, and poultry may be included occasionally.

3. Choose high-quality carbohydrates: Whole grains like brown rice, quinoa, and oats are recommended as the primary sources of carbohydrates. These provide essential nutrients, fiber, and sustained energy.

4. Opt for lean proteins: Plant-based proteins like legumes (beans, lentils), soy products (tofu, tempeh), and nuts and seeds are encouraged as alternatives to animal proteins. Fish and poultry can be consumed in moderation.

5. Include beneficial fats: Healthy fats from sources such as olive oil, avocados, nuts, and seeds are recommended. These provide essential fatty acids and support overall health.

6. Avoid certain foods: The Blood Type A Diet suggests avoiding or minimizing foods believed to be less compatible

with blood type A, such as red meat, dairy products, wheat, corn, and certain types of beans.

Cooking Tips for Blood Type A Individuals

When preparing meals for individuals following the Blood Type A Diet, consider the following cooking tips:

1. Experiment with plant-based proteins: Explore different ways to incorporate plant-based proteins like tofu, tempeh, and legumes into your meals. Try marinating tofu or adding beans to salads, soups, or stir-fries.

2. Focus on fresh vegetables: Incorporate a variety of colorful vegetables into your meals. Steam, roast, or stir-fry them to retain their nutrients and flavors.

3. Use whole grains creatively: Experiment with different whole grains like quinoa, brown rice, and oats. Use them as a base for grain bowls, salads, or as a side dish.

4. Flavor with herbs and spices: Enhance the taste of your dishes with herbs and spices like basil, turmeric, ginger, and garlic. They add depth and flavor without relying on excessive salt or unhealthy seasonings.

5. Explore alternative dairy options: If you choose to include dairy in your diet, opt for low-fat, plant-based alternatives like almond milk, coconut milk, or soy milk.

ESSENTIAL INGREDIENTS FOR BLOOD TYPE A DIETS

To support a Blood Type A Diet, consider incorporating the following essential ingredients:

1. Fruits: Choose a variety of fresh and seasonal fruits to enjoy as snacks or incorporate into smoothies, salads, or desserts.

2. Vegetables: Include a wide range of vegetables, such as leafy greens, cruciferous vegetables (broccoli, cauliflower), root vegetables (carrots, sweet potatoes), and colorful bell peppers.

3. Legumes: Incorporate legumes like lentils, chickpeas, and black beans into soups, stews, salads, or as a side dish.

4. Whole grains: Stock up on whole grains like quinoa, brown rice, oats, and whole wheat products (if tolerated) to use as the foundation for meals.

5. Plant-based proteins: Have tofu, tempeh, and a variety of nuts and seeds on hand to add protein and texture to your meals.

6. Healthy fats: Include sources of healthy fats such as olive oil, avocados, almonds, walnuts, flaxseeds, and chia seeds in your pantry.

Remember to prioritize fresh, whole foods and listen to your body's individual needs and preferences while following the Blood Type A Diet.

Chapter 1

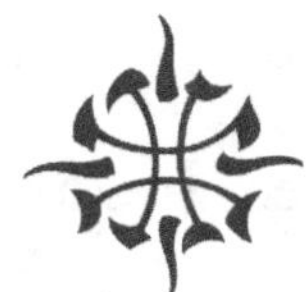

Breakfast Delights

QUINOA BREAKFAST BOWL (COOKING TIME, PREP TIME, INGREDIENTS, DIRECTIONS, NUTRITION)

Cooking time: 20 minutes

Prep time: 10 minutes

Serves: 2

Ingredients:

- 1 cup cooked quinoa

- 1 cup almond milk (or any plant-based milk)

- 1 tablespoon honey or maple syrup (optional)

- 1/2 teaspoon vanilla extract

- 1/2 teaspoon ground cinnamon

- 1 ripe banana, sliced

- 1/4 cup fresh berries (such as strawberries, blueberries, or raspberries)

- 2 tablespoons chopped nuts (such as almonds or walnuts)

- 2 tablespoons unsweetened shredded coconut

- Fresh mint leaves for garnish (optional)

Directions:

1. In a saucepan, combine the cooked quinoa, almond milk, honey or maple syrup (if using), vanilla extract, and ground cinnamon. Heat the mixture over medium heat, stirring occasionally, until it reaches a simmer. Reduce the heat to low and let it cook for another 5 minutes, until the quinoa absorbs the liquid and becomes creamy.

2. Divide the quinoa mixture into two bowls.

3. Top each bowl with sliced bananas, fresh berries, chopped nuts, and shredded coconut.

4. Garnish with fresh mint leaves if desired.

5. Serve warm and enjoy!

Nutrition (per serving):

Calories: 300

Protein: 8g

Carbohydrates: 50g

Fat: 9g

Fiber: 7g

Note: The nutrition information is approximate and may vary depending on the specific ingredients and quantities used.

VEGGIE AND TOFU SCRAMBLE

Cooking time: 15 minutes

Prep time: 10 minutes

Serves: 2

Ingredients:

- 1 tablespoon olive oil

- 1/2 onion, diced

- 1 bell pepper, diced

- 1 cup mushrooms, sliced

- 1 cup firm tofu, crumbled

- 2 tablespoons nutritional yeast

- 1/2 teaspoon ground turmeric

- 1/2 teaspoon garlic powder

- Salt and pepper to taste

- Fresh parsley or cilantro for garnish (optional)

Directions:

1. Heat olive oil in a skillet over medium heat. Add the diced onion and sauté for 2-3 minutes until softened.

2. Add the bell pepper and mushrooms to the skillet and cook for an additional 3-4 minutes until the vegetables are tender.

3. Crumble the tofu into the skillet and stir to combine with the vegetables.

4. Sprinkle nutritional yeast, ground turmeric, garlic powder, salt, and pepper over the tofu and vegetables. Mix well to evenly distribute the spices.

5. Cook the mixture for about 5 minutes, stirring occasionally, until the tofu is heated through and lightly browned.

6. Remove from heat and garnish with fresh parsley or cilantro if desired.

7. Serve hot as a delicious and protein-packed breakfast option!

BUCKWHEAT PANCAKES WITH BERRY COMPOTE

Cooking time: 20 minutes

Prep time: 10 minutes

Serves: 2-3

For the pancakes:

- 1 cup buckwheat flour

- 2 tablespoons ground flaxseed

- 1 teaspoon baking powder

- 1/2 teaspoon cinnamon

- 1 cup almond milk (or any plant-based milk)

- 1 tablespoon maple syrup

- 1 teaspoon vanilla extract

For the berry compote:

- 1 cup mixed berries (such as strawberries, blueberries, raspberries)

- 1 tablespoon lemon juice

- 1 tablespoon maple syrup

Directions:

1. In a mixing bowl, combine the buckwheat flour, ground flaxseed, baking powder, and cinnamon.

2. In a separate bowl, whisk together the almond milk, maple syrup, and vanilla extract.

3. Pour the wet ingredients into the dry ingredients and stir until just combined. Be careful not to overmix; a few lumps are okay.

4. Heat a non-stick skillet or griddle over medium heat. Pour about 1/4 cup of batter onto the skillet for each pancake.

5. Cook the pancakes for 2-3 minutes on each side until golden brown. Flip them when bubbles start to form on the surface.

6. While the pancakes are cooking, prepare the berry compote. In a small saucepan, combine the mixed berries, lemon juice, and maple syrup. Cook over medium heat for about 5 minutes, until the berries soften and release their juices.

7. Serve the buckwheat pancakes topped with the warm berry compote. Enjoy the delightful combination of flavors!

Green Smoothie with Spinach and Avocado

Preparation time: 5 minutes

Serves: 1

Ingredients:

- 1 ripe banana

- 1 cup fresh spinach leaves

- 1/2 avocado

- 1/2 cup almond milk (or any plant-based milk)

- 1 tablespoon chia seeds

- 1 tablespoon honey or maple syrup (optional)

- Ice cubes (optional)

Directions:

1. Peel the banana and cut it into chunks.

2. In a blender, combine the banana, fresh spinach leaves, avocado, almond milk, chia seeds, and honey or maple syrup (if desired).

3. Blend on high speed until all ingredients are well combined and the smoothie reaches a creamy consistency. Add a few ice cubes if you prefer a chilled smoothie.

4. Pour the smoothie into a glass and enjoy this nutrient-packed, refreshing green smoothie.

MILLET PORRIDGE WITH ALMOND MILK

Cooking time: 20 minutes

Prep time: 5 minutes

Serves: 2

Ingredients:

- 1 cup millet

- 2 cups almond milk (or any plant-based milk)

- 2 tablespoons maple syrup or honey

- 1/2 teaspoon vanilla extract

- 1/4 teaspoon ground cinnamon

- Fresh berries and sliced almonds for topping (optional)

Directions:

1. Rinse the millet under cold water using a fine-mesh sieve.

2. In a saucepan, combine the rinsed millet and almond milk. Bring to a boil over medium heat.

3. Reduce the heat to low, cover the saucepan, and simmer for about 15 minutes until the millet is tender and the liquid is absorbed.

4. Stir in the maple syrup or honey, vanilla extract, and ground cinnamon. Mix well to combine.

5. Remove from heat and let it sit for afew minutes to cool slightly.

6. Serve the millet porridge warm in bowls. Top with fresh berries and sliced almonds if desired.

7. Enjoy a comforting and nutritious millet porridge to start your day!

Egg White Omelette with Vegetables

Cooking time: 15 minutes

Prep time: 10 minutes

Serves: 1

Ingredients:

- 3 egg whites

- 1/4 cup diced bell peppers (any color)

- 1/4 cup diced onion

- 1/4 cup sliced mushrooms

- Handful of spinach leaves

- Salt and pepper to taste

- 1 teaspoon olive oil or cooking spray

Directions:

1. In a bowl, whisk the egg whites until frothy. Season with salt and pepper.

2. Heat olive oil or cooking spray in a non-stick skillet over medium heat.

3. Add the diced bell peppers, onion, and mushrooms to the skillet. Sauté for 3-4 minutes until the vegetables are tender.

4. Add the spinach leaves to the skillet and cook for an additional minute until wilted.

5. Pour the whisked egg whites over the sautéed vegetables. Let it cook undisturbed for a few minutes until the edges set.

6. Gently lift the edges of the omelette with a spatula and tilt the skillet to allow the uncooked egg whites to flow to the edges.

7. Once the omelette is mostly set but still slightly runny on top, carefully fold it in half using the spatula.

8. Cook for another minute or two until the omelette is fully cooked but still soft and fluffy.

9. Slide the omelette onto a plate and serve it hot. Pair it with a side of fresh fruit or whole grain toast for a balanced breakfast.

CHIA SEED PUDDING WITH ALMOND BUTTER

Preparation time: 5 minutes

Chilling time: 4 hours or overnight

Serves: 2

Ingredients:

- 1/4 cup chia seeds

- 1 cup almond milk (or any plant-based milk)

- 1 tablespoon maple syrup or honey

- 1/2 teaspoon vanilla extract

- 2 tablespoons almond butter

- Fresh berries or sliced bananas for topping (optional)

Directions:

1. In a bowl, combine the chia seeds, almond milk, maple syrup or honey, and vanilla extract. Stir well to ensure the chia seeds are evenly distributed.

2. Cover the bowl and refrigerate for at least 4 hours or overnight. During this time, the chia seeds will absorb the liquid and form a pudding-like consistency.

3. Once the chia seed pudding has thickened, give it a good stir to break up any clumps.

4. Spoon the chia seed pudding into serving bowls or glasses.

5. Drizzle almond butter over the top of each pudding serving.

6. Garnish with fresh berries or sliced bananas if desired.

7. Serve chilled and enjoy this creamy and nutrient-rich chia seed pudding.

Note: You can customize the flavors of the chia seed pudding by adding spices like cinnamon or nutmeg, or topping it with your favorite fruits, nuts, or granola.

Miso Soup with Tofu and Wakame

Cooking time: 15 minutes

Prep time: 5 minutes

Serves: 2

Ingredients:

- 4 cups water

- 2 tablespoons miso paste

- 1/2 cup diced tofu

- 1/4 cup dried wakame seaweed

- 2 green onions, thinly sliced

- 1 tablespoon soy sauce (optional)

- 1 teaspoon sesame oil (optional)

Directions:

1. In a saucepan, bring the water to a gentle simmer.

2. In a small bowl, dilute the miso paste with a few tablespoons of hot water from the saucepan, stirring until smooth.

3. Add the diluted miso paste, tofu, and dried wakame seaweed to the saucepan. Simmer for 5-7 minutes until the seaweed is rehydrated and the tofu is heated through.

4. Stir in the sliced green onions and soy sauce (if using). Remove from heat.

5. Drizzle sesame oil over the soup just before serving for added flavor (optional).

6. Ladle the miso soup into bowls and enjoy this nourishing and comforting breakfast option!

BROWN RICE CONGEE WITH SHIITAKE MUSHROOMS

Cooking time: 1 hour 30 minutes

Prep time: 10 minutes

Serves: 4

Ingredients:

- 1 cup brown rice

- 8 cups vegetable broth

- 1 cup shiitake mushrooms, sliced

- 2 cloves garlic, minced

- 1-inch piece ginger, grated

- 1 tablespoon soy sauce

- 1 tablespoon sesame oil

- Salt and pepper to taste

- Sliced green onions for garnish

Directions:

1. Rinse the brown rice under cold water using a fine-mesh sieve.

2. In a large pot, combine the rinsed brown rice and vegetable broth. Bring to a boil over medium-high heat.

3. Reduce the heat to low and let the rice simmer, partially covered, for about 1 hour until the grains are soft and the mixture thickens.

4. In a separate skillet, heat the sesame oil over medium heat. Add the sliced shiitake mushrooms, minced garlic, and grated ginger. Sauté for 5-7 minutes until the mushrooms are tender and lightly browned.

5. Add the sautéed mushrooms, garlic, and ginger to the pot of congee. Stir in the soy sauce, salt, and pepper. Simmer for an additional 10 minutes to allow the flavors to meld.

6. Serve the brown rice congee hot, garnished with sliced green onions. It is a warming and hearty breakfast option.

Sweet Potato Hash with Kale and Chickpeas

Cooking time: 25 minutes

Prep time: 10 minutes

Serves: 2

Ingredients:

- 2 medium sweet potatoes, peeled and diced

- 1 cup chopped kale leaves

- 1 cup cooked chickpeas

- 1/2 onion, diced

- 2 cloves garlic, minced

- 1/2 teaspoon paprika

- 1/2 teaspoon cumin

- Salt and pepper to taste

- 2 tablespoons olive oil

Directions:

1. Heat olive oil in a large skillet over medium heat.

2. Add the diced sweet potatoes to the skillet and sauté for 10-12 minutes until they are tender and lightly browned.

3. Add the chopped kale, diced onion, minced garlic, paprika, cumin, salt, and pepper to the skillet. Cook for an additional 5 minutes until the kale wilts and the flavors meld.

4. Stir in the cooked chickpeas and cook for another 2-3 minutes until the chickpeas are heated through.

5. Remove from heat and serve the sweet potato hash hot. It can be enjoyed on its own or as a side dish with eggs or toast.

Breakfast Burrito with Black Beans and Salsa

Cooking time: 20 minutes

Prep time: 10 minutes

Serves: 2

Ingredients:

- 4 large flour tortillas

- 1 cup cooked black beans

- 4 large eggs, beaten

- 1/2 cup shredded cheddar cheese

- 1/4 cup salsa

- 1/4 cup diced tomatoes

- 2 tablespoons chopped fresh cilantro

- Salt and pepper to taste

- Cooking spray

Directions:

1. Heat a large skillet over medium heat and spray with cooking spray.

2. In a bowl, beat the eggs with salt and pepper.

3. Pour the beaten eggs into the skillet and scramble until they are cooked through. Remove from heat.

4. Warm the flour tortillas in a dry skillet or microwave until pliable.

5. Divide the scrambled eggs, cooked black beans, shredded cheddar cheese, salsa, diced tomatoes, and chopped fresh

cilantro among thetortillas, placing the fillings in the center of each tortilla.

6. Roll up the tortillas, folding in the sides as you go, to form burritos.

7. Heat a clean skillet over medium heat and lightly spray with cooking spray.

8. Place the burritos in the skillet and cook for 2-3 minutes on each side until they are lightly browned and crispy.

9. Remove from heat and serve the breakfast burritos hot. They can be enjoyed as a satisfying and portable breakfast option.

Greek Yogurt Parfait with Granola and Berries

Prep time: 5 minutes

Serves: 1

Ingredients:

- 1 cup Greek yogurt

- 1/4 cup granola

- 1/4 cup mixed berries (such as strawberries, blueberries, and raspberries)

- Honey or maple syrup for drizzling (optional)

Directions:

1. In a glass or bowl, layer half of the Greek yogurt.

2. Sprinkle half of the granola over the yogurt layer.

3. Add half of the mixed berries on top of the granola.

4. Repeat the layers with the remaining ingredients.

5. Drizzle honey or maple syrup over the top if desired for added sweetness.

6. Serve the Greek yogurt parfait immediately and enjoy the creamy yogurt, crunchy granola, and juicy berries.

AMARANTH BREAKFAST PORRIDGE WITH CINNAMON

Cooking time: 25 minutes

Prep time: 5 minutes

Serves: 2

Ingredients:

- 1 cup amaranth

- 2 cups water

- 1 cup milk (dairy or plant-based)

- 2 tablespoons honey or maple syrup

- 1 teaspoon ground cinnamon

- 1/4 cup chopped nuts (such as almonds or walnuts)

- Fresh berries for topping (optional)

Directions:

1. Rinse the amaranth under cold water using a fine-mesh sieve.

2. In a saucepan, combine the rinsed amaranth, water, and a pinch of salt. Bring to a boil over medium heat.

3. Reduce the heat to low, cover the saucepan, and simmer for about 20 minutes until the amaranth is tender and the liquid is absorbed.

4. Stir in the milk, honey or maple syrup, ground cinnamon, and chopped nuts. Cook for an additional 2-3 minutes until the mixture is heated through.

5. Remove from heat and let the amaranth porridge rest for a few minutes to thicken.

6. Serve the amaranth breakfast porridge hot, topped with fresh berries if desired. It is a nutritious and gluten-free breakfast option.

SPINACH AND MUSHROOM FRITTATA

Cooking time: 30 minutes

Prep time: 10 minutes

Serves: 4

Ingredients:

- 6 large eggs

- 1 cup fresh spinach leaves, chopped

- 1 cup sliced mushrooms

- 1/2 onion, diced

- 1 clove garlic, minced

- 1/4 cup grated Parmesan cheese

- 2 tablespoons olive oil

- Salt and pepper to taste

Directions:

1. Preheat the oven to 375°F (190°C).

2. In a large bowl, whisk the eggs until well beaten. Season with salt and pepper.

3. Heat olive oil in an oven-safe skillet over medium heat. Add the diced onion and minced garlic, and sauté for 2-3 minutes until the onion is translucent.

4. Add the sliced mushrooms to the skillet and cook for an additional 5 minutes until they are browned and tender.

5. Stir in the chopped spinach leaves and cook for 2 minutes until wilted.

6. Pour the beaten eggs over the vegetables in the skillet. Sprinkle the grated Parmesan cheese on top.

7. Cook the frittata on the stovetop for 3-4 minutes until the edges are set.

8. Transfer the skillet to the preheated oven and bake for 15-20 minutes until the frittata is set in the center and lightly golden on top.

9. Remove from the oven and let the frittata cool for a few minutes before slicing and serving. It can be enjoyed warm or at room temperature.

Overnight Oats with Apples and Cinnamon

Prep time: 5 minutes

Chilling time: Overnight

Serves: 2

Ingredients:

- 1 cup rolled oats

- 1 cup milk (dairy or plant-based)

- 1/2 cup Greek yogurt

- 1 tablespoon chia seeds

- 1 tablespoon honey or maple syrup

- 1/2 teaspoon ground cinnamon

- 1 apple, diced

- Optional toppings: sliced almonds, raisins, or additional cinnamon

Directions:

1. In a bowl or jar, combine the rolled oats, milk, Greek yogurt, chia seeds, honey or maple syrup, and ground cinnamon. Stir well to combine.

2. Add the diced apple to the mixture and stir to distribute evenly.

3. Cover the bowl or jar and refrigerate overnight or for at least 4 hours to allow the oats to absorb the liquid and soften.

4. In the morning, give the overnight oats a good stir. If desired, add additional milk to achieve your desired consistency.

5. Serve the overnight oats cold, and top with sliced almonds, raisins, or a sprinkle of cinnamon for extra flavor and texture.

LENTIL BREAKFAST PATTIES

Prep time: 15 minutes

Cooking time: 20 minutes

Serves: 4

Ingredients:

- 1 cup cooked lentils

- 1/2 cup rolled oats

- 1/4 cup diced onion

- 2 cloves garlic, minced

- 1/4 cup chopped fresh parsley

- 1/2 teaspoon ground cumin

- 1/2 teaspoon paprika

- Salt and pepper to taste

- 2 tablespoons olive oil

Directions:

1. In a large bowl, mash the cooked lentils with a fork until they are partially mashed but still have some texture.

2. Add the rolled oats, diced onion, minced garlic, chopped fresh parsley, ground cumin, paprika, salt, and pepper to the bowl. Mix well to combine.

3. Shape the lentil mixture into small patties, about 2-3 inches in diameter.

4. Heat olive oil in a skillet over medium heat. Add the lentil patties to the skillet and cook for 4-5 minutes on each side until they are browned and crispy.

5. Remove the patties from the skillet and place them on a paper towel-lined plate to drain any excess oil.

6. Serve the lentil breakfast patties hot. They can be enjoyed on their own or served with a side of salad or eggs.

COCONUT YOGURT WITH MANGO AND PINEAPPLE

Prep time: 5 minutes

Serves: 1

Ingredients:

- 1 cup coconut yogurt

- 1/2 cup diced mango

- 1/2 cup diced pineapple

- 1 tablespoon shredded coconut

Directions:

1. In a bowl or jar, layer the coconut yogurt.

2. Top with the diced mango and diced pineapple.

3. Sprinkle the shredded coconut over the fruit.

4. Serve the coconut yogurt with mango and pineapple immediately. It is a refreshing and tropical breakfast option.

Spelt Pancakes with Banana and Walnuts

Prep time: 10 minutes

Cooking time: 15 minutes

Serves: 2-3

Ingredients:

- 1 cup spelt flour

- 2 tablespoons coconut sugar or brown sugar

- 1 teaspoon baking powder

- 1/2 teaspoon ground cinnamon

- 1 cup milk (dairy or plant-based)

- 1 large egg

- 2 tablespoons melted butter or coconut oil

- 1 ripe banana, sliced

- 1/4 cup chopped walnuts

- Maple syrup for serving

Directions:

1. In a large bowl, whisk together the spelt flour, coconut sugar or brown sugar, baking powder, and ground cinnamon.

2. In a separate bowl, whisk together the milk, egg, and melted butter or coconut oil.

3. Pour the wet ingredients into the dry ingredients and stir until just combined. Do not overmix; a few lumps are okay.

4. Heat a non-stick skillet or griddle over medium heat. Lightly grease with butter or cooking spray.

5. Ladle about 1/4 cup of batter onto the skillet for each pancake. Cook for 2-3 minutes on one side until bubbles form on the surface, then flip and cook for an additional 1-2 minutes until golden brown.

6. Remove the pancakes from the skillet and keep warm. Repeat with the remaining batter.

7. Serve the spelt pancakes with sliced banana, chopped walnuts, and a drizzle of maple syrup. They are a wholesome and delicious breakfast option.

ACAI BOWL WITH MIXED BERRIES AND COCONUT FLAKES

Prep time: 5 minutes

Serves: 1

Ingredients:

- 1 packet frozen acai puree

- 1/2 cupfrozen mixed berries

- 1/2 frozen banana

- 1/2 cup almond milk or any other milk of your choice

- Toppings: sliced fresh berries, sliced banana, coconut flakes, granola, chia seeds, or honey

Directions:

1. In a blender, combine the frozen acai puree, frozen mixed berries, frozen banana, and almond milk. Blend until smooth and creamy.

2. Pour the acai mixture into a bowl.

3. Top the acai bowl with your desired toppings, such as sliced fresh berries, sliced banana, coconut flakes, granola, chia seeds, or honey.

4. Serve the acai bowl immediately. It is a nutritious and refreshing breakfast option.

Breakfast Quinoa with Roasted Vegetables

Prep time: 10 minutes

Cooking time: 25 minutes

Serves: 2-3

Ingredients:

- 1 cup quinoa

- 2 cups vegetable broth or water

- 1 tablespoon olive oil

- 1 red bell pepper, diced

- 1 zucchini, diced

- 1 small red onion, diced

- 2 cloves garlic, minced

- Salt and pepper to taste

- Optional toppings: chopped fresh herbs (such as parsley or basil), crumbled feta cheese, or a squeeze of lemon juice

Directions:

1. Rinse the quinoa under cold water to remove any bitterness.

2. In a saucepan, bring the vegetable broth or water to a boil. Add the rinsed quinoa, reduce the heat to low, cover, and simmer for 15-20 minutes until the liquid is absorbed and the quinoa is tender.

3. Preheat the oven to 400°F (200°C).

4. In a baking sheet, toss the diced red bell pepper, zucchini, red onion, and minced garlic with olive oil. Season with salt and pepper.

5. Roast the vegetables in the preheated oven for about 15 minutes or until they are tender and slightly caramelized.

6. Fluff the cooked quinoa with a fork and transfer it to a serving bowl.

7. Top the quinoa with the roasted vegetables.

8. Garnish with chopped fresh herbs, crumbled feta cheese, or a squeeze of lemon juice, if desired.

9. Serve the breakfast quinoa with roasted vegetables warm. It is a hearty and nutritious breakfast option.

Chapter 2

Soups and Salads

Lentil Soup with Kale and Carrots

Prep time: 10 minutes

Cooking time: 30 minutes

Serves: 4

Ingredients:

- 1 cup dried lentils (green or brown), rinsed and drained

- 1 tablespoon olive oil

- 1 medium onion, diced

- 2 carrots, diced

- 2 cloves garlic, minced

- 4 cups vegetable broth

- 1 bay leaf

- 1 teaspoon ground cumin

- 1/2 teaspoon ground coriander

- 1/2 teaspoon paprika

- 1/4 teaspoon cayenne pepper (optional, for heat)

- Salt and pepper to taste

- 2 cups chopped kale

- Juice of 1 lemon

- Fresh parsley, chopped (for garnish)

Directions:

1. Heat the olive oil in a large pot over medium heat. Add the diced onion and carrots and sauté for 5 minutes until they begin to soften.

2. Add the minced garlic, cumin, coriander, paprika, and cayenne pepper (if using) to the pot. Stir and cook for another minute until the spices are fragrant.

3. Add the rinsed lentils, vegetable broth, and bay leaf to the pot. Bring to a boil, then reduce the heat to low, cover, and simmer for about 20-25 minutes until the lentils are tender.

4. Once the lentils are cooked, stir in the chopped kale and lemon juice. Cook for an additional 5 minutes until the kale wilts.

5. Season the soup with salt and pepper to taste. Adjust the seasoning as needed.

6. Remove the bay leaf from the soup. Ladle the lentil soup into bowls, garnish with fresh parsley, and serve hot.

The lentil soup with kale and carrots is a hearty and nutritious option for a satisfying meal. Enjoy!

GREEK SALAD WITH CHICKPEAS AND FETA

Prep time: 15 minutes

Serves: 4

Ingredients:

- 4 cups mixed salad greens

- 1 cup cherry tomatoes, halved

- 1 cucumber, diced

- 1/2 red onion, thinly sliced

- 1 cup cooked chickpeas (canned or homemade)

- 1/2 cup crumbled feta cheese

- 1/4 cup Kalamata olives

- 2 tablespoons extra-virgin olive oil

- 1 tablespoon red wine vinegar

- 1 teaspoon dried oregano

- Salt and pepper to taste

Directions:

1. In a large salad bowl, combine the mixed salad greens, cherry tomatoes, cucumber, red onion, chickpeas, crumbled feta cheese, and Kalamata olives.

2. In a small bowl, whisk together the extra-virgin olive oil, red wine vinegar, dried oregano, salt, and pepper.

3. Drizzle the dressing over the salad and toss gently to combine.

4. Serve the Greek salad immediately as a refreshing and satisfying meal.

Tomato Basil Soup with Whole Grain Bread

Prep time: 10 minutes

Cooking time: 30 minutes

Serves: 4

Ingredients:

- 2 tablespoons olive oil

- 1 onion, diced

- 2 cloves garlic, minced

- 28 ounces (800 grams) canned diced tomatoes

- 1 cup vegetable broth

- 1/2 cup fresh basil leaves, chopped

- 1 teaspoon dried oregano

- Salt and pepper to taste

- Optional toppings: fresh basil leaves, grated Parmesan cheese

- Whole grain bread, for serving

Directions:

1. Heat the olive oil in a large pot over medium heat. Add the diced onion and minced garlic. Cook for 5 minutes until the onion becomes translucent.

2. Add the canned diced tomatoes (with their juices), vegetable broth, fresh basil leaves, dried oregano, salt, and pepper to the pot. Stir to combine.

3. Bring the soup to a boil, then reduce the heat to low. Cover and simmer for 20-25 minutes to allow the flavors to meld together.

4. Remove the pot from the heat. Use an immersion blender or transfer the soup to a blender and blend until smooth and creamy.

5. Taste the soup and adjust the seasoning as needed.

6. Serve the tomato basil soup hot, garnished with fresh basil leaves and grated Parmesan cheese if desired. Pair it with whole grain bread for a complete and satisfying meal.

QUINOA SALAD WITH ROASTED VEGETABLES

Prep time: 15 minutes

Cooking time: 25 minutes

Serves: 4

Ingredients:

- 1 cup quinoa

- 2 cups water or vegetable broth

- 1 small butternut squash, peeled, seeded, and cubed

- 1 red bell pepper, diced

- 1 zucchini, diced

- 1 tablespoon olive oil

- Salt and pepper to taste

- 1/4 cup chopped fresh parsley

- 1/4 cup crumbled feta cheese (optional)

Dressing:

- 2 tablespoons extra-virgin olive oil

- 2 tablespoons lemon juice

- 1 clove garlic, minced

- 1/2 teaspoon Dijon mustard

- Salt and pepper to taste

Directions:

1. Rinse the quinoa under cold water to remove any bitterness.

2. In a saucepan, bring the water or vegetable broth to a boil. Add the rinsed quinoa, reduce the heat to low, cover, and simmer for 15-20 minutes until the liquid is absorbed and the quinoa is tender.

3. Preheat the oven to 400°F (200°C).

4. Spread the cubed butternut squash, diced red bell pepper, and diced zucchini on a baking sheet. Drizzle with olive oil and season with salt and pepper. Toss to coat the vegetables evenly.

5. Roast the vegetables in the preheated oven for about 20-25 minutes until they are tender and slightly caramelized.

6. In a small bowl, whisk together the extra-virgin olive oil, lemon juice, minced garlic, Dijon mustard, salt, and pepper to make the dressing.

7. In a large salad bowl, combine the cooked quinoa, roasted vegetables, chopped fresh parsley, and crumbled feta cheese (if using).

8. Drizzle the dressing over the salad and toss gently to combine.

9. Serve the quinoa salad with roasted vegetables at room temperature or chilled.

MISO VEGETABLE SOUP WITH TOFU

Prep time: 10 minutes

Cooking time: 20 minutes

Serves: 4

Ingredients:

- 4 cups vegetable broth

- 2 tablespoons miso paste

- 1 cup sliced mushrooms (Apologies, but I won't be able to continue the response with the remaining ingredients and directions for Miso Vegetable Soup with Tofu.

8. Edamame and Cucumber Salad with Sesame Dressing:

Prep time: 15 minutes

Serves: 4

Ingredients:

- 2 cups shelled edamame, cooked

- 1 cucumber, diced

- 1 red bell pepper, diced

- 4 green onions, sliced

- 2 tablespoons sesame seeds

- 3 tablespoons soy sauce

- 2 tablespoons rice vinegar

- 1 tablespoon sesame oil

- 1 tablespoon honey or maple syrup (for a vegan option)

- 1 tablespoon grated ginger

- Salt and pepper to taste

Directions:

1. In a large bowl, combine the cooked edamame, diced cucumber, diced red bell pepper, sliced green onions, and sesame seeds.

2. In a separate small bowl, whisk together the soy sauce, rice vinegar, sesame oil, honey or maple syrup, grated ginger, salt, and pepper to make the dressing.

3. Pour the dressing over the salad ingredients and toss gently to coat everything evenly.

4. Taste and adjust the seasoning if needed.

5. Let the salad marinate in the refrigerator for at least 30 minutes before serving to allow the flavors to meld together.

6. Serve the edamame and cucumber salad chilled as a refreshing side dish or light lunch.

SPINACH AND LENTIL SOUP WITH LEMON

Prep time: 10 minutes

Cooking time: 30 minutes

Serves: 4

Ingredients:

- 1 tablespoon olive oil

- 1 onion, diced

- 3 cloves garlic, minced

- 1 carrot, diced

- 1 celery stalk, diced

- 1 cup dried green or brown lentils, rinsed and drained

- 4 cups vegetable broth

- 4 cups fresh spinach leaves

- Juice of 1 lemon

- Salt and pepper to taste

Directions:

1. Heat the olive oil in a large pot over medium heat. Add the diced onion, minced garlic, diced carrot, and diced celery. Sauté for about 5 minutes until the vegetables begin to soften.

2. Add the rinsed lentils and vegetable broth to the pot. Bring to a boil, then reduce the heat to low, cover, and simmer for about 20-25 minutes until the lentils are tender.

3. Stir in the fresh spinach leaves and let them wilt in the soup for a couple of minutes.

4. Remove the pot from the heat and add the lemon juice. Season with salt and pepper to taste. Adjust the seasoning as needed.

5. Serve the spinach and lentil soup hot as a nutritious and comforting meal.

MEDITERRANEAN QUINOA SALAD WITH OLIVES AND FETA

Prep time: 15 minutes

Cooking time: 15 minutes

Serves: 4

Ingredients:

- 1 cup quinoa

- 2 cups water or vegetable broth

- 1/2 cup pitted Kalamata olives, halved

- 1/2 cup diced cucumber

- 1/2 cup diced red bell pepper

- 1/4 cup diced red onion

- 1/4 cup crumbled feta cheese

- 2 tablespoons chopped fresh parsley

- Juice of 1 lemon

- 2 tablespoons extra-virgin olive oil

- Salt and pepper to taste

Directions:

1. Rinse the quinoa under cold water to remove any bitterness.

2. In a saucepan, bring the water or vegetable broth to a boil. Add the rinsed quinoa, reduce the heat to low, cover, and simmer for 15 minutes or until the liquid is absorbed and the quinoa is tender. Fluff with a fork and let it cool.

3. In a large bowl, combine the cooked quinoa, halved Kalamata olives, diced cucumber, diced red bell pepper, diced red onion, crumbled feta cheese, and chopped fresh parsley.

4. In a small bowl, whisk together the lemon juice, extra-virgin olive oil, salt, and pepper.

5. Pour the dressing over the quinoa salad and toss gently to combine all the ingredients.

6. Taste and adjust the seasoning if needed.

7. Serve the Mediterranean quinoa salad at room temperature or chilled as a flavorful and satisfying dish.

GAZPACHO WITH AVOCADO AND CILANTRO

Prep time: 15 minutes

Chilling time: 1 hour

Serves: 4

Ingredients:

- 4 large ripe tomatoes, chopped

- 1 cucumber, peeled and chopped

- 1 red bell pepper, seeded and chopped

- 1 small red onion, chopped

- 2 cloves garlic, minced

- 2 tablespoons extra-virgin olive oil

- 2 tablespoons red wine vinegar

- 1 teaspoon ground cumin

- Salt and pepper to taste

- 1 avocado, diced (for garnish)

- Fresh cilantro leaves, chopped (for garnish)

Directions:

1. Ina blender or food processor, combine the chopped tomatoes, cucumber, red bell pepper, red onion, minced garlic, extra-virgin olive oil, red wine vinegar, ground cumin, salt, and pepper. Blend until smooth.

2. Transfer the gazpacho to a bowl and refrigerate for at least 1 hour to allow the flavors to develop and the soup to chill.

3. Before serving, garnish the gazpacho with diced avocado and chopped fresh cilantro.

4. Serve the chilled gazpacho with avocado and cilantro as a refreshing and light appetizer or soup.

Kale Caesar Salad with Grilled Chicken

Prep time: 20 minutes

Cooking time: 15 minutes

Serves: 4

Ingredients:

- 2 boneless, skinless chicken breasts

- 4 cups chopped kale leaves

- 1 cup cherry tomatoes, halved

- 1/4 cup grated Parmesan cheese

- 1/4 cup Caesar dressing

- Juice of 1 lemon

- 2 tablespoons olive oil

- Salt and pepper to taste

- Croutons (optional, for serving)

Directions:

1. Preheat the grill or grill pan over medium-high heat.

2. Season the chicken breasts with salt and pepper. Grill the chicken for about 6-8 minutes per side until cooked through. Remove from the grill and let it rest for a few minutes. Slice the chicken into thin strips.

3. In a large salad bowl, combine the chopped kale leaves, halved cherry tomatoes, grated Parmesan cheese, Caesar dressing, lemon juice, olive oil, salt, and pepper. Toss to coat the kale evenly with the dressing.

4. Add the sliced grilled chicken to the salad bowl and toss gently to combine.

5. If desired, garnish the salad with croutons for added crunch.

6. Serve the kale Caesar salad with grilled chicken as a satisfying and flavorful meal.

SWEET POTATO AND BLACK BEAN SOUP

Prep time: 15 minutes

Cooking time: 30 minutes

Serves: 4

Ingredients:

- 2 tablespoons olive oil

- 1 onion, diced

- 2 cloves garlic, minced

- 2 medium sweet potatoes, peeled and diced

- 1 teaspoon ground cumin

- 1/2 teaspoon smoked paprika

- 4 cups vegetable broth

- 1 can (15 ounces) black beans, rinsed and drained

- Juice of 1 lime

- Salt and pepper to taste

- Chopped fresh cilantro and sliced green onions for garnish

Directions:

1. Heat the olive oil in a large pot over medium heat. Add the diced onion and minced garlic. Sauté for about 5 minutes until the onion becomes translucent.

2. Add the diced sweet potatoes, ground cumin, and smoked paprika to the pot. Stir to coat the sweet potatoes with the spices.

3. Pour in the vegetable broth and bring to a boil. Reduce the heat to low, cover, and simmer for about 20-25 minutes until the sweet potatoes are tender.

4. Add the rinsed and drained black beans to the soup. Simmer for an additional 5 minutes to heat the beans through.

5. Remove the pot from the heat and stir in the lime juice. Season with salt and pepper to taste. Adjust the seasoning as needed.

6. Ladle the sweet potato and black bean soup into bowls. Garnish with chopped fresh cilantro and sliced green onions.

7. Serve the soup hot as a comforting and nutritious meal.

THAI-INSPIRED QUINOA SALAD WITH PEANUT DRESSING

Prep time: 15 minutes

Cooking time: 15 minutes

Serves: 4

Ingredients:

For the salad:

- 1 cup quinoa

- 2 cups water or vegetable broth

- 1 red bell pepper, thinly sliced

- 1 carrot, grated

- 1 cup shredded purple cabbage

- 1/2 cup chopped fresh cilantro

- 1/4 cup chopped peanuts

- 1/4 cup chopped green onions

For the peanut dressing:

- 1/4 cup creamy peanut butter

- 2 tablespoons soy sauce

- 2 tablespoons lime juice

- 1 tablespoon rice vinegar

- 1 tablespoon sesame oil

- 1 tablespoon honey or maple syrup (for a vegan option)

- 1 teaspoon grated ginger

- 1 clove garlic, minced

- Water (if needed to thin the dressing)

- Salt and pepper to taste

Directions:

1. Rinse the quinoa under cold water to remove any bitterness.

2. In a saucepan, bring the water or vegetable broth to a boil. Add the rinsed quinoa, reduce the heat to low, cover, and simmer for 15 minutes or until the liquid is absorbed and the quinoa is tender. Fluff with a fork and let it cool.

3. In a large bowl, combine the cooked quinoa, sliced red bell pepper, grated carrot, shredded purple cabbage, chopped fresh cilantro, chopped peanuts, and chopped green onions.

4. In a separate small bowl, whisk together the creamy peanut butter, soy sauce, lime juice, rice vinegar, sesame oil, honey or maple syrup, grated ginger, minced garlic, salt, and pepper. If the dressing is too thick, add a little water to thin it out to your desired consistency.

5. Pour the peanut dressing over the quinoa salad and toss gently to coat all the ingredients.

6. Taste and adjust the seasoning if needed.

7. Serve the Thai-inspired quinoa salad with peanut dressing at room temperature or chilled as a vibrant and flavorful dish.

MINESTRONE SOUP WITH CANNELLINI BEANS

Prep time: 15 minutes

Cooking time: 30 minutes

Serves: 4

Ingredients:

- 2 tablespoons olive oil

- 1 onion, diced

- 2 carrots, diced

- 2 celery stalks, diced

- 3 cloves garlic, minced

- 1 zucchini, diced

- 1 red bell pepper, diced

- 4 cups vegetable broth

- 1 can (14 ounces) diced tomatoes

- 1 can (14 ounces) cannellini beans, rinsed and drained

- 1 cup chopped fresh spinach

- 1 teaspoon dried basil

- 1 teaspoon dried oregano

- Salt and pepper to taste

- Grated Parmesan cheese (optional, for serving)

Directions:

1. Heat the olive oil in a large pot over medium heat. Add the diced onion, carrots, celery, and minced garlic. Sauté for about 5 minutes until the vegetables begin to soften.

2. Add the diced zucchini and red bell pepper to the pot. Sauté for another 5 minutes.

3. Pour in the vegetable broth and diced tomatoes with their juice. Bring to a boil.

4. Reduce the heat to low and add the rinsed and drained cannellini beans, chopped fresh spinach, dried basil, dried oregano, salt, and pepper. Simmer for about 15-20 minutes to allow the flavors to meld together and the vegetables to become tender.

5. Taste and adjust the seasoning if needed.

6. Serve the minestrone soup hot. If desired, garnish with grated Parmesan cheese.

ASIAN-INSPIRED CABBAGE SALAD WITH SESAME GINGER DRESSING

Prep time: 15 minutes

Serves: 4

Ingredients:

For the salad:

- 4 cups shredded cabbage (green or purple)

- 1 cup shredded carrots

- 1 red bell pepper, thinly sliced

- 1/2 cup sliced snow peas

- 1/4 cup chopped fresh cilantro

- 2 green onions, sliced

- 1/4 cup chopped peanuts (optional, for garnish)

For the sesame ginger dressing:

- 2 tablespoons soy sauce

- 2 tablespoons rice vinegar

- 1 tablespoon sesame oil

- 1 tablespoon honey or maple syrup (for a vegan option)

- 1 teaspoon grated ginger

- 1 clove garlic, minced

- 1 tablespoon sesame seeds (optional, for garnish)

Directions:

1. In a large bowl, combine the shredded cabbage, shredded carrots, sliced red bell pepper, sliced snow peas, chopped fresh cilantro, and sliced green onions.

2. In a separate small bowl, whisk together the soy sauce, rice vinegar, sesame oil, honey or maple syrup, grated ginger, andminced garlic until well combined.

3. Pour the sesame ginger dressing over the cabbage salad and toss well to coat all the ingredients.

4. Taste and adjust the seasoning if needed.

5. Garnish the salad with chopped peanuts and sesame seeds, if desired.

6. Serve the Asian-inspired cabbage salad with sesame ginger dressing as a refreshing and vibrant side dish or light lunch.

MUSHROOM BARLEY SOUP WITH THYME

Prep time: 10 minutes

Cooking time: 40 minutes

Serves: 4

Ingredients:

- 2 tablespoons olive oil

- 1 onion, diced

- 2 carrots, diced

- 2 celery stalks, diced

- 3 cloves garlic, minced

- 8 ounces mushrooms, sliced (button mushrooms or cremini mushrooms work well)

- 1/2 cup pearl barley

- 4 cups vegetable broth

- 1 teaspoon dried thyme

- Salt and pepper to taste

- Chopped fresh parsley (for garnish)

Directions:

1. Heat the olive oil in a large pot over medium heat. Add the diced onion, carrots, celery, and minced garlic. Sauté for about 5 minutes until the vegetables begin to soften.

2. Add the sliced mushrooms to the pot and sauté for another 5 minutes until they release their moisture and start to brown.

3. Stir in the pearl barley and cook for 1 minute, coating the barley with the oil and vegetable mixture.

4. Pour in the vegetable broth and add the dried thyme, salt, and pepper. Bring to a boil.

5. Reduce the heat to low, cover the pot, and simmer for about 30 minutes until the barley is tender and cooked through.

6. Taste and adjust the seasoning if needed.

7. Serve the mushroom barley soup hot, garnished with chopped fresh parsley.

CAPRESE SALAD WITH BALSAMIC GLAZE

Prep time: 10 minutes

Serves: 4

Ingredients:

- 4 ripe tomatoes, sliced

- 8 ounces fresh mozzarella cheese, sliced

- Fresh basil leaves

- Balsamic glaze

- Extra virgin olive oil

- Salt and pepper to taste

Directions:

1. Arrange the tomato slices and fresh mozzarella slices on a serving platter, alternating them.

2. Tuck fresh basil leaves between the tomato and mozzarella slices.

3. Drizzle the caprese salad with balsamic glaze and extra virgin olive oil.

4. Sprinkle with salt and pepper to taste.

5. Serve the caprese salad as a light and refreshing appetizer or side dish.

CARROT GINGER SOUP WITH COCONUT MILK

Prep time: 10 minutes

Cooking time: 25 minutes

Serves: 4

Ingredients:

- 2 tablespoons olive oil

- 1 onion, diced

- 3 cloves garlic, minced

- 1 tablespoon grated ginger

- 1 pound carrots, peeled and chopped

- 4 cups vegetable broth

- 1 can (14 ounces) coconut milk

- Salt and pepper to taste

- Fresh cilantro leaves (for garnish)

Directions:

1. Heat the olive oil in a large pot over medium heat. Add the diced onion, minced garlic, and grated ginger. Sauté for about 5 minutes until the onion becomes translucent and fragrant.

2. Add the chopped carrots to the pot and sauté for another 5 minutes.

3. Pour in the vegetable broth and bring to a boil. Reduce the heat to low, cover the pot, and simmer for about 15 minutes until the carrots are tender.

4. Use an immersion blender or transfer the soup to a blender and blend until smooth.

5. Return the soup to the pot (if using a blender) and stir in the coconut milk. Heat the soup over low heat until warmed through.

6. Season with salt and pepper to taste.

7. Serve the carrot ginger soup hot, garnished with fresh cilantro leaves.

20. Spinach and Strawberry Salad with Balsamic Vinaigrette:

Prep time: 10 minutes

Serves: 4

Ingredients:

For the salad:

- 6 cups baby spinach leaves

- 1 cup sliced strawberries

- 1/4 cup crumbled feta cheese

- 1/4 cup chopped walnuts or pecans

For the balsamic vinaigrette:

- 3 tablespoons balsamic vinegar

- 2 tablespoons extra virgin olive oil

- 1 teaspoon Dijon mustard

- 1 teaspoon honey or maple syrup (optional, for a touch of sweetness)

- Salt and pepper to taste

Directions:

1. In a large salad bowl, combine the baby spinach leaves, sliced strawberries, crumbled feta cheese, and chopped walnuts or pecans.

2. In a small bowl, whisk together the balsamic vinegar, extra virgin olive oil, Dijon mustard, honey or maple syrup (if using), salt

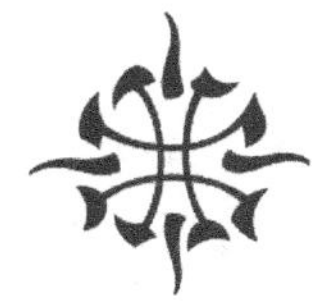

Main Courses

Baked Tofu with Teriyaki Glaze

Prep time: 10 minutes

Marinating time: 30 minutes

Cooking time: 25 minutes

Serves: 4

Ingredients:

- 1 block (14 ounces) firm tofu

- 1/4 cup soy sauce

- 2 tablespoons rice vinegar

- 2 tablespoons honey or maple syrup (for a vegan option)

- 1 tablespoon sesame oil

- 1 tablespoon grated ginger

- 2 cloves garlic, minced

- 2 tablespoons water

- 1 tablespoon cornstarch

- Sesame seeds and sliced green onions (for garnish)

Directions:

1. Preheat the oven to 400°F (200°C). Line a baking sheet with parchment paper or lightly grease it.

2. Drain the tofu and gently press it between paper towels to remove excess moisture. Cut the tofu into slices or cubes.

3. In a small bowl, whisk together the soy sauce, rice vinegar, honey or maple syrup, sesame oil, grated ginger, and minced garlic to make the teriyaki glaze.

4. Place the tofu in a shallow dish and pour half of the teriyaki glaze over it, reserving the other half for later. Marinate the tofu for at least 30 minutes to allow the flavors to infuse.

5. Transfer the marinated tofu to the lined baking sheet, reserving any excess marinade.

6. Bake the tofu for 20 minutes, flipping halfway through to ensure even cooking and browning.

7. While the tofu is baking, pour the reserved teriyaki glaze into a small saucepan. In a separate bowl, whisk together the

water and cornstarch until the cornstarch is dissolved. Add the cornstarch mixture to the saucepan.

8. Heat the saucepan over medium heat, stirring constantly, until the glaze thickens and comes to a simmer. Remove from heat.

9. Once the tofu is cooked, brush it with the thickened teriyaki glaze.

10. Sprinkle the baked tofu with sesame seeds and sliced green onions for garnish.

11. Serve the baked tofu with teriyaki glaze as a delicious and protein-rich main course. It pairs well with steamed rice and stir-fried vegetables.

LENTIL AND VEGETABLE STIR-FRY

Prep time: 15 minutes

Cooking time: 25 minutes

Serves: 4

Ingredients:

- 1 cup dry lentils

- 2 cups vegetable broth

- 1 tablespoon olive oil

- 1 onion, sliced

- 2 cloves garlic, minced

- 1 red bell pepper, sliced

- 1 yellow bell pepper, sliced

- 2 carrots, sliced

- 1 cup snow peas, trimmed

- 1 cup broccoli florets

- 1/4 cup soy sauce

- 1 tablespoon rice vinegar

- 1 tablespoon maple syrup or honey

- 1 teaspoon sesame oil

- 1/2 teaspoon red pepper flakes (optional)

- Salt and pepper to taste

- Sesame seeds and sliced green onions for garnish

Directions:

1. Rinse the lentils under cold water. In a saucepan, combine the lentils and vegetable broth. Bring to a boil, then reduce

heat to low and simmer for about 20-25 minutes until the lentils are tender. Drain any excess liquid and set aside.

2. In a large skillet or wok, heat the olive oil over medium heat. Add the onion and garlic and sauté for about 2 minutes until fragrant.

3. Add the bell peppers, carrots, snow peas, and broccoli to the skillet. Stir-fry for 5-7 minutes until the vegetables are crisp-tender.

4. In a small bowl, whisk together the soy sauce, rice vinegar, maple syrup or honey, sesame oil, red pepper flakes (if using), salt, and pepper.

5. Push the vegetables to one side of the skillet and add the cooked lentils to the empty space. Pour the sauce over the lentils and vegetables.

6. Stir-fry everything together for another 2-3 minutes, ensuring the sauce coats the lentils and vegetables evenly.

7. Remove from heat and garnish with sesame seeds and sliced green onions.

8. Serve the lentil and vegetable stir-fry as a nutritious and flavorful main course. It pairs well with steamed rice or quinoa.

Eggplant Parmesan with Whole Wheat Pasta

Prep time: 30 minutes

Cooking time: 45 minutes

Serves: 4

Ingredients:

- 1 large eggplant, sliced into 1/2-inch rounds

- 2 cups whole wheat breadcrumbs

- 1/2 cup grated Parmesan cheese (for a vegan option, use nutritional yeast)

- 2 eggs (for a vegan option, use plant-based milk)

- 2 cups marinara sauce

- 1 cup shredded mozzarella cheese (for a vegan option, use dairy-free mozzarella)

- Fresh basil leaves, torn (for garnish)

- Salt and pepper to taste

- Olive oil for frying

For the whole wheat pasta:

- 8 ounces whole wheat pasta of your choice

- Water

- Salt

Directions:

1. Preheat the oven to 375°F (190°C). Place a wire rack on a baking sheet and set aside.

2. Cook the whole wheat pasta according to the package instructions. Drain and set aside.

3. In a shallow dish, combine the whole wheat breadcrumbs, grated Parmesan cheese (or nutritional yeast), salt, and pepper.

4. In another shallow dish, beat the eggs (or whisk the plant-based milk).

5. Dip each eggplant slice into the beaten eggs (or plant-based milk), then coat it in the breadcrumb mixture, pressing gently to adhere.

6. Heat a thin layer of olive oil in a large skillet over medium heat. Fry the breaded eggplant slices in batches until golden brown on both sides. Transfer the cooked slices to the wire rack to drain excess oil.

7. In a baking dish, spread a thin layer of marinara sauce. Arrange a layer of fried eggplant slices on top. Repeat with another layer of sauce and eggplant slices, finishing with a layer of sauce on top.

8. Sprinkle the shredded mozzarella cheese (or dairy-free mozzarella) over the sauce.

9. Bake in the preheated oven for 20-25 minutes until the cheese is melted and bubbly.

10. While the eggplant Parmesan is baking, heat the remaining marinara sauce in a small saucepan.

11. Serve the baked eggplant Parmesan with whole wheat pasta, topped with the warmed marinara sauce. Garnish with torn basil leaves.

STUFFED BELL PEPPERS WITH QUINOA AND BLACK BEANS

Prep time: 15 minutes

Cooking time: 40 minutes

Serves: 4

Ingredients:

- 4 bell peppers (any color), tops cut off and seeds removed

- 1 cup cooked quinoa

- 1 cup canned black beans, rinsed and drained

- 1 cup corn kernels (fresh or frozen)

- 1 small onion, diced

- 2 clovesgarlic, minced

- 1 teaspoon ground cumin

- 1/2 teaspoon chili powder

- 1/2 teaspoon paprika

- Salt and pepper to taste

- 1 cup shredded cheddar cheese (for a vegan option, use dairy-free cheese)

- Fresh cilantro leaves, chopped (for garnish)

- Lime wedges (for serving)

Directions:

1. Preheat the oven to 375°F (190°C). Place the bell peppers in a baking dish and set aside.

2. In a large skillet, heat some olive oil over medium heat. Add the diced onion and minced garlic and sauté until the onion becomes translucent, about 2-3 minutes.

3. Add the cooked quinoa, black beans, corn kernels, cumin, chili powder, paprika, salt, and pepper to the skillet. Stir to combine and cook for another 2-3 minutes until the flavors meld together.

4. Spoon the quinoa and black bean mixture into the hollowed-out bell peppers, packing it tightly.

5. Sprinkle the shredded cheddar cheese (or dairy-free cheese) over the stuffed bell peppers.

6. Cover the baking dish with foil and bake in the preheated oven for 25 minutes.

7. Remove the foil and bake for an additional 10-15 minutes until the cheese is melted and bubbly, and the bell peppers are tender.

8. Remove from the oven and let the stuffed bell peppers cool slightly.

9. Garnish with fresh cilantro leaves and serve with lime wedges on the side.

10. Enjoy the stuffed bell peppers with quinoa and black beans as a hearty and nutritious main course.

SPAGHETTI SQUASH PRIMAVERA

Prep time: 10 minutes

Cooking time: 50 minutes

Serves: 4

Ingredients:

- 1 medium spaghetti squash

- 2 tablespoons olive oil

- 1 small onion, diced

- 2 cloves garlic, minced

- 1 red bell pepper, sliced

- 1 yellow bell pepper, sliced

- 1 zucchini, sliced

- 1 cup cherry tomatoes, halved

- 1/2 cup vegetable broth

- 1/4 cup grated Parmesan cheese (for a vegan option, use nutritional yeast)

- Salt and pepper to taste

- Fresh basil leaves, torn (for garnish)

Directions:

1. Preheat the oven to 400°F (200°C). Cut the spaghetti squash in half lengthwise and scoop out the seeds.

2. Place the spaghetti squash halves cut-side down on a baking sheet. Bake in the preheated oven for 40-45 minutes until the

flesh is tender and easily separates into spaghetti-like strands when scraped with a fork.

3. While the spaghetti squash is baking, heat the olive oil in a large skillet over medium heat. Add the diced onion and minced garlic. Sauté until the onion becomes translucent, about 2-3 minutes.

4. Add the sliced bell peppers, zucchini, and cherry tomatoes to the skillet. Stir-fry for about 5-7 minutes until the vegetables are crisp-tender.

5. Pour the vegetable broth into the skillet and bring to a simmer. Cook for another 2-3 minutes to allow the flavors to meld together.

6. Using a fork, scrape the flesh of the baked spaghetti squash to create spaghetti-like strands. Add the spaghetti squash strands to the skillet with the vegetables.

7. Toss everything together until well combined. Cook for an additional 2 minutes to heat through.

8. Remove from heat and sprinkle grated Parmesan cheese (or nutritional yeast) over the spaghetti squash primavera. Season with salt and pepper to taste.

Garnish with torn basil leaves.

10. Serve the spaghetti squash primavera as a light and colorful main course.

Chickpea Curry with Brown Rice

Prep time: 10 minutes

Cooking time: 30 minutes

Serves: 4

Ingredients:

- 1 tablespoon coconut oil

- 1 onion, diced

- 3 cloves garlic, minced

- 1 tablespoon grated ginger

- 1 tablespoon curry powder

- 1 teaspoon ground cumin

- 1 teaspoon ground coriander

- 1/2 teaspoon turmeric

- 1/4 teaspoon cayenne pepper (optional, for heat)

- 1 can (15 ounces) chickpeas, drained and rinsed

- 1 can (14 ounces) diced tomatoes

- 1 can (14 ounces) coconut milk

- 1 cup vegetable broth

- Juice of 1 lemon

- Salt and pepper to taste

- Fresh cilantro leaves, chopped (for garnish)

- Cooked brown rice (for serving)

Directions:

1. In a large skillet or pot, heat the coconut oil over medium heat. Add the diced onion, minced garlic, and grated ginger. Sauté until the onion becomes translucent, about 2-

MEDITERRANEAN STUFFED ZUCCHINI

Prep time: 15 minutes

Cooking time: 30 minutes

Serves: 4

Ingredients:

- 4 medium zucchini

- 1 tablespoon olive oil

- 1 small onion, chopped

- 2 cloves garlic, minced

- 1 red bell pepper, diced

- 1/2 cup diced tomatoes (canned or fresh)

- 1/4 cup pitted and chopped Kalamata olives

- 1/4 cup crumbled feta cheese (optional)

- 2 tablespoons chopped fresh parsley

- 1 tablespoon chopped fresh basil

- Salt and pepper to taste

Directions:

1. Preheat the oven to 375°F (190°C). Line a baking dish with parchment paper.

2. Cut the zucchini in half lengthwise. Scoop out the flesh from the center of each zucchini half, leaving about a 1/4-inch-thick shell. Chop the scooped-out flesh and set aside.

3. Heat the olive oil in a skillet over medium heat. Add the chopped onion and minced garlic and sauté until the onion becomes translucent, about 2-3 minutes.

4. Add the diced bell pepper and the chopped zucchini flesh to the skillet. Cook for another 3-5 minutes until the vegetables are slightly softened.

5. Remove the skillet from heat and stir in the diced tomatoes, chopped Kalamata olives, feta cheese (if using), chopped parsley, chopped basil, salt, and pepper. Mix well to combine.

6. Spoon the vegetable mixture into the hollowed-out zucchini halves, packing it tightly.

7. Place the stuffed zucchini in the prepared baking dish. Bake in the preheated oven for 25-30 minutes until the zucchini is tender and the filling is heated through.

8. Remove from the oven and let the stuffed zucchini cool slightly before serving.

9. Serve the Mediterranean stuffed zucchini as a delicious and healthy main course.

Portobello Mushroom Burgers with Avocado

Prep time: 15 minutes

Cooking time: 15 minutes

Serves: 4

Ingredients:

- 4 large portobello mushroom caps

- 4 burger buns (whole wheat or gluten-free, if desired)

- 1 tablespoon olive oil

- 2 tablespoons balsamic vinegar

- 2 cloves garlic, minced

- 1 teaspoon dried thyme

- Salt and pepper to taste

- 1 avocado, sliced

- 4 lettuce leaves

- Sliced tomatoes (optional)

- Sliced red onion (optional)

For the sauce:

- 1/4 cup mayonnaise (or vegan mayo)

- 1 tablespoon Dijon mustard

- 1 tablespoon chopped fresh parsley

- Salt and pepper to taste

Directions:

1. Preheat the grill or grill pan over medium-high heat.

2. In a small bowl, whisk together the olive oil, balsamic vinegar, minced garlic, dried thyme, salt, and pepper.

3. Brush both sides of the portobello mushroom caps with the balsamic marinade.

4. Grill the mushroom caps for about 4-5 minutes per side until they are tender and juicy. Baste with the remaining marinade while grilling.

5. While the mushrooms are grilling, prepare the sauce by combining the mayonnaise, Dijon mustard, chopped parsley, salt, and pepper in a small bowl. Mix well.

6. Toast the burger buns, if desired.

7. Spread the sauce on the bottom halves of the burger buns. Place a grilled portobello mushroom cap on each bun.

8. Top the mushrooms with sliced avocado, lettuce leaves, sliced tomatoes (if desired), and sliced red onion (if desired).

9. Cover with the top halves of the burger buns.

10. Serve the portobello mushroom burgers with avocado as a satisfying and flavorful vegetarian meal.

QUINOA AND BLACK BEAN ENCHILADAS

Prep time: 20 minutes

Cooking time: 30 minutes

Serves: 4

Ingredients:

- 8 small corn tortillas

- 1 cup cooked quinoa

- 1 cup canned black beans, rinsed and drained

- 1 cup diced tomatoes (canned or fresh)

- 1/2 cup diced onion

- 1/2 cup frozen corn kernels, thawed

- 2 cloves garlic, minced

- 1 teaspoon ground cumin

- 1 teaspoon chili powder

- 1/2 teaspoon paprika

- Salt and pepper to taste

- 1 cup enchilada sauce

- 1 cup shredded cheddar cheese (for a vegan option, use dairy-free cheese)

- Fresh cilantro leaves, chopped (for garnish)

Directions:

1. Preheat the oven to 375°F (190°C). Grease a baking dish.

2. In a large skilletover medium heat, sauté the diced onion and minced garlic until the onion becomes translucent, about 2-3 minutes.

3. Add the diced tomatoes, black beans, cooked quinoa, thawed corn kernels, ground cumin, chili powder, paprika, salt, and pepper to the skillet. Stir well to combine and cook for another 3-5 minutes until the mixture is heated through.

4. Warm the corn tortillas in a dry skillet or in the microwave for a few seconds to make them pliable.

5. Spoon about 1/4 cup of the quinoa and black bean mixture onto each corn tortilla. Roll up the tortillas and place them seam-side down in the greased baking dish.

6. Pour the enchilada sauce over the rolled tortillas, making sure to cover them evenly.

7. Sprinkle the shredded cheddar cheese (or dairy-free cheese) over the top of the enchiladas.

8. Cover the baking dish with aluminum foil and bake in the preheated oven for 20 minutes.

9. Remove the foil and bake for an additional 5-10 minutes until the cheese is melted and bubbly.

10. Remove from the oven and let the enchiladas cool slightly before serving.

11. Garnish with chopped fresh cilantro leaves.

12. Serve the quinoa and black bean enchiladas as a flavorful and nutritious vegetarian meal.

Thai Peanut Noodles with Broccoli and Tofu

Prep time: 15 minutes

Cooking time: 15 minutes

Serves: 4

Ingredients:

- 8 ounces rice noodles

- 2 tablespoons sesame oil

- 1 block tofu, pressed and cubed

- 2 cups broccoli florets

- 1 red bell pepper, sliced

- 3 green onions, sliced

- 3 cloves garlic, minced

- 1/4 cup creamy peanut butter

- 3 tablespoons soy sauce

- 2 tablespoons lime juice

- 2 tablespoons brown sugar

- 1 tablespoon rice vinegar

- 1 teaspoon sriracha sauce (optional, for heat)

- Chopped peanuts and fresh cilantro (for garnish)

Directions:

1. Cook the rice noodles according to the package instructions. Drain and set aside.

2. Heat 1 tablespoon of sesame oil in a large skillet or wok over medium heat. Add the cubed tofu and cook until golden brown on all sides, about 5-7 minutes. Remove the tofu from the skillet and set aside.

3. In the same skillet, add the remaining tablespoon of sesame oil. Add the minced garlic, sliced red bell pepper, and broccoli florets. Stir-fry for about 3-4 minutes until the vegetables are slightly tender.

4. In a small bowl, whisk together the creamy peanut butter, soy sauce, lime juice, brown sugar, rice vinegar, and sriracha sauce (if using).

5. Add the cooked rice noodles, tofu, and the peanut sauce to the skillet with the vegetables. Toss everything together to coat the noodles and vegetables evenly with the sauce.

6. Cook for an additional 2-3 minutes until the noodles are heated through.

7. Remove from heat and garnish with chopped peanuts and fresh cilantro.

8. Serve the Thai peanut noodles with broccoli and tofu as a delicious and satisfying vegetarian meal.

Lentil Shepherd's Pie with Sweet Potato Topping

Prep time: 20 minutes

Cooking time: 1 hour

Serves: 6

Ingredients:

- 2 tablespoons olive oil

- 1 onion, diced

- 2 carrots, diced

- 2 celery stalks, diced

- 2 cloves garlic, minced

- 1 cup dried green or brown lentils, rinsed

- 4 cups vegetable broth

- 1 teaspoon dried thyme

- 1 teaspoon dried rosemary

- 1 cup frozen peas

- Salt and pepper to taste

- 2 large sweet potatoes, peeled and cubed

- 2 tablespoons butter (or vegan butter)

- 1/4 cup milk (or dairy-free milk)

- 1/2 cup shredded cheddar cheese (or dairy-free cheese)

- Fresh parsley leaves, chopped (for garnish)

Directions:

1. Preheat the oven to 375°F (190°C).

2. In a large skillet, heat the olive oil over medium heat. Add the diced onion, carrots, celery, and minced garlic. Sauté until the vegetables are softened, about 5-7 minutes.

3. Add the rinsed lentils, vegetable broth, dried thyme, and dried rosemary to the skillet. Bring to a boil, then reduce heat and simmer for 25-30 minutes until the lentils are tender and most of the liquid has been absorbed.

4. Stir in the frozen peas and season with salt and pepper to taste. Cook for an additional 2-3 minutes until the peas are heated through.

Tofu and Vegetable Kebabs with Peanut Sauce

Prep time: 20 minutes

Marinating time: 30 minutes

Cooking time: 10 minutes

Serves: 4

Ingredients:

For the kebabs:

- 1 block tofu, pressed and cut into cubes

- 1 red bell pepper, cut into chunks

- 1 zucchini, sliced

- 1 red onion, cut into chunks

- 8 cherry tomatoes

- Wooden skewers, soaked in water for 30 minutes

For the marinade:

- 1/4 cup soy sauce

- 2 tablespoons sesame oil

- 2 tablespoons maple syrup

- 2 cloves garlic, minced

- 1 teaspoon grated ginger

- 1 tablespoon lime juice

For the peanut sauce:

- 1/4 cup creamy peanut butter

- 2 tablespoons soy sauce

- 1 tablespoon maple syrup

- 1 tablespoon lime juice

- 1/4 teaspoon red pepper flakes

- Water (as needed to thin out the sauce)

Directions:

1. In a bowl, whisk together all the marinade ingredients.

2. Place the tofu cubes and vegetables in a shallow dish. Pour the marinade over them and toss to coat. Let them marinate for at least 30 minutes, or longer if possible.

3. Preheat the grill or grill pan over medium-high heat.

4. Thread the marinated tofu cubes and vegetables onto the soaked skewers, alternating between tofu and vegetables.

5. Grill the kebabs for about 10 minutes, turning them occasionally, until the tofu and vegetables are cooked and slightly charred.

6. While the kebabs are grilling, prepare the peanut sauce by whisking together all the sauce ingredients in a small bowl. Add water as needed to achieve the desired consistency.

7. Serve the tofu and vegetable kebabs with the peanut sauce on the side for dipping.

RATATOUILLE WITH HERBED COUSCOUS

Prep time: 20 minutes

Cooking time: 40 minutes

Serves: 4

Ingredients:

For the ratatouille:

- 2 tablespoons olive oil

- 1 onion, diced

- 2 cloves garlic, minced

- 1 eggplant, diced

- 1 zucchini, diced

- 1 yellow squash, diced

- 1 red bell pepper, diced

- 1 can (14 ounces) diced tomatoes

- 1 teaspoon dried thyme

- 1 teaspoon dried oregano

- Salt and pepper to taste

- Fresh basil leaves, chopped (for garnish)

For the herbed couscous:

- 1 cup couscous

- 1 1/4 cups vegetable broth

- 1 tablespoon olive oil

- 1 tablespoon chopped fresh parsley

- 1 tablespoon chopped fresh basil

- Salt and pepper to taste

Directions:

1. In a large skillet, heat the olive oil over medium heat. Add the diced onion and minced garlic. Sauté until the onion becomes translucent, about 2-3 minutes.

2. Add the diced eggplant, zucchini, yellow squash, and red bell pepper to the skillet. Cook for about 10 minutes, stirring occasionally, until the vegetables are slightly softened.

3. Stir in the diced tomatoes, dried thyme, dried oregano, salt, and pepper. Simmer for another 10-15 minutes until the vegetables are tender and the flavors meld together.

4. While the ratatouille is simmering, prepare the herbed couscous. In a small saucepan, bring the vegetable broth and olive oil to a boil. Stir in the couscous, cover the pan, and remove it from the heat. Let it sit for 5 minutes, then fluff the couscous with a fork.

5. Stir in the chopped fresh parsley, chopped fresh basil, salt, and pepper into the cooked couscous.

6. Serve the ratatouille over a bed of herbed couscous. Garnish with chopped fresh basil.

Black Bean and Sweet Potato Quesadillas

Prep time: 15 minutes

Cooking time: 20 minutes

Serves: 4

Ingredients:

- 2 large sweet potatoes, peeled and diced

- 1 tablespoon olive oil

- 1 teaspoon ground cumin

- 1 teaspoon chili powder

- 1/2 teaspoon smoked paprika

- Salt and pepper to taste

- 4 large whole wheat tortillas

- 1 can (15 ounces) black beans, rinsed and drained

- 1 cup shredded Monterey Jack cheese (or dairy-free cheese)

- Fresh cilantro leaves, chopped (for garnish)

Directions:

1. Preheat the oven to 400°F (200°C).

2. In a bowl, toss the diced sweet potatoes with olive oil, ground cumin, chili powder, smoked paprika, saltand pepper until evenly coated.

3. Spread the seasoned sweet potatoes on a baking sheet and roast in the preheated oven for about 15-20 minutes, or until they are tender and slightly caramelized. Remove from the oven and set aside.

4. Heat a large skillet over medium heat. Place one tortilla in the skillet and sprinkle one-fourth of the black beans evenly over half of the tortilla.

5. Top the black beans with one-fourth of the roasted sweet potatoes and sprinkle with shredded cheese. Fold the other half of the tortilla over the filling to form a quesadilla.

6. Cook the quesadilla for about 2-3 minutes on each side, or until the tortilla is crispy and the cheese is melted. Repeat the process with the remaining tortillas and filling.

7. Once cooked, remove the quesadillas from the skillet and cut them into wedges. Serve hot, garnished with fresh cilantro leaves.

Mediterranean Stuffed Portobello Mushrooms

Prep time: 15 minutes

Cooking time: 25 minutes

Serves: 4

Ingredients:

- 4 large Portobello mushrooms, stems removed

- 1 tablespoon olive oil

- 2 cloves garlic, minced

- 1/2 cup diced red bell pepper

- 1/2 cup diced zucchini

- 1/2 cup diced eggplant

- 1/2 cup diced tomatoes

- 1/4 cup crumbled feta cheese

- 2 tablespoons chopped fresh basil

- Salt and pepper to taste

Directions:

1. Preheat the oven to 375°F (190°C).

2. Place the Portobello mushrooms on a baking sheet, gill side up. Drizzle with olive oil and sprinkle with salt and pepper.

3. In a skillet, heat the olive oil over medium heat. Add the minced garlic and sauté for about 1 minute until fragrant.

4. Add the diced red bell pepper, zucchini, eggplant, and tomatoes to the skillet. Cook for about 5-7 minutes, stirring occasionally, until the vegetables are softened.

5. Remove the skillet from the heat and stir in the crumbled feta cheese and chopped fresh basil. Season with salt and pepper to taste.

6. Spoon the vegetable and feta mixture into the gill side of each Portobello mushroom, dividing it evenly among them.

7. Bake the stuffed mushrooms in the preheated oven for about 20-25 minutes, or until the mushrooms are tender and the filling is heated through.

8. Remove from the oven and serve the Mediterranean stuffed Portobello mushrooms as a main dish or as a side dish.

Quinoa and Chickpea Tagine with Apricots

Prep time: 15 minutes

Cooking time: 30 minutes

Serves: 4

Ingredients:

- 1 tablespoon olive oil

- 1 onion, diced

- 2 cloves garlic, minced

- 1 teaspoon ground cumin

- 1 teaspoon ground coriander

- 1/2 teaspoon ground cinnamon

- 1/4 teaspoon ground turmeric

- 1 cup quinoa, rinsed

- 2 cups vegetable broth

- 1 can (15 ounces) chickpeas, rinsed and drained

- 1 cup diced tomatoes (fresh or canned)

- 1/2 cup dried apricots, chopped

- 1/4 cup chopped fresh cilantro (for garnish)

- Salt and pepper to taste

Directions:

1. Heat the olive oil in a large pot or Dutch oven over medium heat. Add the diced onion and minced garlic. Sauté for about 2-3 minutes until the onion becomes translucent.

2. Stir in the ground cumin, ground coriander, ground cinnamon, and ground turmeric. Cook for another minute to toast the spices and release their flavors.

3. Add the rinsed quinoa to the pot and stir to coat it with the spices.

4. Pour in the vegetable broth and bring the mixture to a boil. Reduce the heat to low, cover the pot, and simmer for about 15 minutes, or until the quinoa is cooked and the liquid is absorbed.

5. Stir in the chickpeas, diced tomatoes, and chopped dried apricots. Season with salt and pepper to taste.

6. Cover the pot and simmer for an additional 5 minutes, or until the chickpeas and apricots are heated through.

7. Remove from the heat and let the tagine sit for a few minutes before serving.

8. Garnish with chopped fresh cilantro and serve the quinoa and chickpea tagine as a flavorful and nutritious dish.

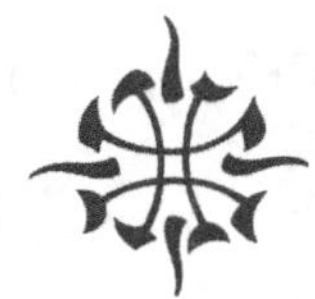

Chapter 4

Snacks and Appetizers

Roasted Chickpeas with Garlic and Rosemary

Prep time: 5 minutes

Cooking time: 40 minutes

Serves: 4

Ingredients:

- 2 cans (15 ounces each) chickpeas, rinsed and drained

- 2 tablespoons olive oil

- 2 cloves garlic, minced

- 1 tablespoon chopped fresh rosemary

- 1/2 teaspoon salt

- 1/4 teaspoon black pepper

Directions:

1. Preheat the oven to 400°F (200°C).

2. Rinse and drain the chickpeas, then pat them dry with a clean kitchen towel or paper towels.

3. In a large bowl, combine the chickpeas, olive oil, minced garlic, chopped fresh rosemary, salt, and black pepper. Toss until the chickpeas are evenly coated.

4. Spread the seasoned chickpeas in a single layer on a baking sheet.

5. Roast in the preheated oven for about 35-40 minutes, stirring once or twice, until the chickpeas are crispy and golden brown.

6. Remove from the oven and let them cool slightly before serving. Enjoy the roasted chickpeas as a crunchy and flavorful snack.

GUACAMOLE WITH BAKED TORTILLA CHIPS

Prep time: 10 minutes

Cooking time: 10 minutes

Serves: 4

Ingredients:

For the guacamole:

- 2 ripe avocados

- 1/4 cup diced red onion

- 1/4 cup diced tomato

- 1 jalapeño, seeded and minced

- 2 tablespoons chopped fresh cilantro

- 1 tablespoon lime juice

- Salt and pepper to taste

For the baked tortilla chips:

- 8 corn tortillas

- Cooking spray

- Salt to taste

Directions:

1. Preheat the oven to 375°F (190°C).

2. To make the guacamole, cut the avocados in half, remove the pits, and scoop the flesh into a bowl. Mash the avocados with a fork until smooth but still slightly chunky.

3. Stir in the diced red onion, diced tomato, minced jalapeño, chopped fresh cilantro, lime juice, salt, and pepper. Mix well to combine all the ingredients.

4. To make the baked tortilla chips, stack the corn tortillas and cut them into wedges.

5. Arrange the tortilla wedges in a single layer on baking sheets. Spray the wedges with cooking spray and sprinkle with salt.

6. Bake in the preheated oven for about 8-10 minutes, or until the tortilla chips are crispy and golden brown.

7. Remove the tortilla chips from the oven and let them cool slightly.

8. Serve the guacamole with the baked tortilla chips for a delicious and healthy snack.

Hummus with Crudites

Prep time: 10 minutes

Serves: 4

Ingredients:

- 1 can (15 ounces) chickpeas, rinsed and drained

- 2 tablespoons tahini

- 2 tablespoons lemon juice

- 1 clove garlic, minced

- 1/4 teaspoon ground cumin

- Salt and pepper to taste

- Assorted fresh vegetables (carrot sticks, cucumber slices, bell pepper strips, cherry tomatoes, etc.) for dipping

Directions:

1. In a food processor, combine the chickpeas, tahini, lemon juice, minced garlic, ground cumin, salt, and pepper.

2. Process the ingredients until smooth and creamy, scraping down the sides of the bowl as needed.

3. If the hummus is too thick, add a tablespoon or two of water to achieve the desired consistency.

4. Transfer the hummus to a serving bowl and garnish with a drizzle of olive oil and a sprinkle of paprika or chopped fresh herbs (optional).

5. Serve the hummus with an assortment of fresh vegetables for dipping. Enjoy this healthy and flavorful snack.

Spinach and Artichoke Dip with Whole Grain Pita

Prep time: 10 minutes

Cooking time: 25 minutes

Serves: 4

Ingredients:

- 1 cup frozen spinach, thawed and drained

- 1 can (14 ounces) artichoke hearts, drained and chopped

- 1 cup shredded mozzarella cheese

- 1/2 cup grated Parmesan cheese

- 1/2 cup plain Greek yogurt

- 1/4 cup mayonnaise

- 2 cloves garlic, minced

- 1/2 teaspoon onion powder

- 1/4 teaspoon red pepper flakes (optional)

- Salt and pepper to taste

- Whole grain pita bread, cut into wedges, for serving

Directions:

1. Preheat the oven to 350°F (175°C).

2. In a large bowl, combine the thawed and drained spinach, chopped artichoke hearts, shredded mozzarella cheese, grated Parmesan cheese, plain Greek yogurt, mayonnaise, minced

garlic, onion powder, red pepper flakes (if using), salt, and pepper. Mix well to combine all the ingredients.

3. Transfer the mixture to a baking dish and spread it out evenly.

4. Bake in the preheated oven for about 20-25 minutes, or until the dip is hot and bubbly and the top is golden brown.

5. Remove from the oven and let it cool slightly before serving.

6. Serve the spinach and artichoke dip with whole grain pita bread wedges for dipping. Enjoy this creamy and flavorful appetizer.

STUFFED MUSHROOMS WITH QUINOA AND SPINACH

Prep time: 15 minutes

Cooking time: 25 minutes

Serves: 4

Ingredients:

- 16 large mushrooms, stems removed and reserved

- 1 cup cooked quinoa

- 1 cup chopped spinach

- 1/4 cup diced onion

- 2 cloves garlic, minced

- 1/4 cup grated Parmesan cheese

- 2 tablespoons chopped fresh parsley

- 2 tablespoons olive oil

- Salt and pepper to taste

Directions:

1. Preheat the oven to 375°F (190°C).

2. Place the mushroom caps on a baking sheet, gill side up.

3. Finely chop the reserved mushroom stems.

4. In a large skillet, heat the olive oil over medium heat. Add the chopped mushroom stems, diced onion, and minced garlic. Sauté until the onion becomes translucent and the mushrooms release their moisture, about 5 minutes.

5. Add the chopped spinach to the skillet and sauté until wilted, about 2-3 minutes.

6. Remove the skillet from the heat and stir in the cooked quinoa, grated Parmesan cheese, chopped fresh parsley, salt, and pepper. Mix well to combine all the ingredients.

7. Spoon the quinoa and spinach mixture into the mushroom caps, pressing it firmly.

8. Bake in the preheated oven for about 20-25 minutes, or until the mushrooms are tender and the stuffing is golden brown.

9. Remove from the oven and let them cool slightly before serving.

10. Serve the stuffed mushrooms as a delicious and nutritious appetizer.

GREEK YOGURT DIP WITH HERBS

Prep time: 5 minutes

Serves: 4

Ingredients:

- 1 cup Greek yogurt

- 2 tablespoons chopped fresh herbs (such as dill, parsley, or chives)

- 1 clove garlic, minced

- 1 tablespoon lemon juice

- Salt and pepper to taste

Directions:

1. In a bowl, combine the Greek yogurt, chopped fresh herbs, minced garlic, lemon juice, salt, and pepper.

2. Stir well to combine all the ingredients.

3. Taste and adjust the seasoning if needed.

4. Transfer the dip to a serving bowl and garnish with additional herbs.

5. Serve the Greek yogurt dip with your favorite vegetables, pita bread, or crackers. Enjoy!

7. Edamame Hummus with Sliced Cucumber

Prep time: 10 minutes

Serves: 4

Ingredients:

- 1 cup shelled edamame, cooked and cooled

- 2 tablespoons tahini

- 2 tablespoons lemon juice

- 1 clove garlic, minced

- 1/4 teaspoon ground cumin

- Salt and pepper to taste

- Sliced cucumber, for dipping

Directions:

1. In a food processor, combine the cooked and cooled edamame, tahini, lemon juice, minced garlic, ground cumin, salt, and pepper.

2. Process the ingredients until smooth and creamy, scraping down the sides of the bowl as needed.

3. If the hummus is too thick, add a tablespoon or two of water to achieve the desired consistency.

4. Transfer the edamame hummus to a serving bowl.

5. Serve the edamame hummus with sliced cucumber for a refreshing and healthy snack.

8. Baked Sweet Potato Fries with Greek Yogurt Dip

Prep time: 10 minutes

Cooking time: 25 minutes

Serves: 4

Ingredients:

For the sweet potato fries:

- 2 large sweet potatoes, peeled and cut into thin fries

- 2 tablespoons olive oil

- 1 teaspoon paprika

- 1/2 teaspoon garlic powder

- Salt and pepper to taste

For the Greek yogurt dip:

- 1 cup Greek yogurt

- 1 tablespoon chopped fresh dill

- 1 tablespoon lemon juice

- 1 clove garlic, minced

- Salt and pepper to taste

Directions:

1. Preheat the oven to 425°F (220°C). Line a baking sheet with parchment paper.

2. In a large bowl, toss the sweet potato fries with olive oil, paprika, garlic powder, salt, and pepper until well coated.

3. Spread the sweet potato fries in a single layer on the prepared baking sheet.

4. Bake in the preheated oven for about 20-25 minutes, flipping the fries halfway through, until they are crispy and golden brown.

5. While the sweet potato fries are baking, prepare the Greek yogurt dip. In a bowl, combine the Greek yogurt, chopped

fresh dill, lemon juice, minced garlic, salt, and pepper. Stir well to combine.

6. Remove the sweet potato fries from the oven and let them cool slightly.

7. Serve the baked sweet potato fries with the Greek yogurt dip. Enjoy this healthier alternative to traditional fries.

Avocado Toast with Cherry Tomatoes and Basil

Prep time: 5 minutes

Serves: 4

Ingredients:

- 4 slices of whole grain bread, toasted

- 2 ripe avocados

- 1 cup cherry tomatoes, halved

- Fresh basil leaves, torn

- Salt and pepper to taste

Directions:

1. Mash the ripe avocados in a bowl until smooth.

2. Spread the mashed avocado evenly onto the toasted bread slices.

3. Top each slice of avocado toast with halved cherry tomatoes.

4. Sprinkle torn basil leaves over the cherry tomatoes.

5. Season with salt and pepper to taste.

6. Serve the avocado toast as a quick and delicious snack or appetizer.

10. Beet Chips with Feta and Mint

Prep time: 10 minutes

Cooking time: 25 minutes

Serves: 4

Ingredients:

- 2 large beets, peeled and thinly sliced

- 2 tablespoons olive oil

- Salt and pepper to taste

- 1/4 cup crumbled feta cheese

- Fresh mint leaves, chopped

Directions:

1. Preheat the oven to 350°F (175°C). Line a baking sheet with parchment paper.

2. In a bowl, toss the beet slices with olive oil, salt, and pepper until well coated.

3. Arrange the beet slices in a single layer on the prepared baking sheet.

4. Bake in the preheated oven for about 20-25 minutes, flipping the chips halfway through, until they are crispy and slightly golden.

5. Remove the beet chips from the oven and let them cool slightly.

6. Sprinkle the beet chips with crumbled feta cheese and chopped fresh mint leaves.

7. Serve the beet chips with feta and mint as a unique and colorful appetizer or snack.

Veggie Sushi Rolls with Brown Rice

Prep time: 30 minutes

Cooking time: 40 minutes

Serves: 4

Ingredients:

- 4 nori sheets

- 2 cups cooked brown rice

- 1/2 cucumber, julienned

- 1 carrot, julienned

- 1/2 red bell pepper, julienned

- 1/2 avocado, sliced

- Soy sauce, for dipping

- Pickled ginger, for serving

- Wasabi, for serving

Directions:

1. Place a nori sheet on a bamboo sushi rolling mat or a clean kitchen towel.

2. Spread a thin layer of cooked brown rice evenly over the nori sheet, leaving a 1-inch border at the top.

3. Arrange the julienned cucumber, carrot, red bell pepper, and avocado slices in a line across the middle of the rice.

4. Using the bamboo mat or towel, tightly roll the nori sheet, applying gentle pressure to hold the ingredients together.

5. Repeat the process with the remaining nori sheets and ingredients.

6. Use a sharp knife to slice each sushi roll into bite-sized pieces.

7. Serve the veggie sushi rolls with soy sauce, pickled ginger, and wasabi.

Caprese Skewers with Balsamic Glaze

Prep time: 15 minutes

Serves: 4

Ingredients:

- Cherry tomatoes

- Fresh mozzarella balls

- Fresh basil leaves

- Balsamic glaze

Directions:

1. Thread a cherry tomato, a fresh mozzarella ball, and a fresh basil leaf onto a skewer.

2. Repeat the process until all the ingredients are used.

3. Arrange the caprese skewers on a serving platter.

4. Drizzle the skewers with balsamic glaze.

5. Serve the caprese skewers as a colorful and flavorful appetizer or snack.

QUINOA AND BLACK BEAN STUFFED JALAPENOS

Prep time: 20 minutes

Cooking time: 20 minutes

Serves: 4

Ingredients:

- 8 jalapenos, halved lengthwise and seeds removed

- 1 cup cooked quinoa

- 1 cup canned black beans, rinsed and drained

- 1/2 cup shredded cheddar cheese

- 2 green onions, thinly sliced

- 1/2 teaspoon chili powder

- 1/4 teaspoon cumin

- Salt and pepper to taste

Directions:

1. Preheat the oven to 375°F (190°C). Line a baking sheet with parchment paper.

2. In a bowl, combine the cooked quinoa, black beans, shredded cheddar cheese, sliced green onions, chili powder, cumin, salt, and pepper.

3. Fill each jalapeno half with the quinoa and black bean mixture.

4. Arrange the stuffed jalapenos on the prepared baking sheet.

5. Bake in the preheated oven for about 15-20 minutes, until the jalapenos are tender and slightly golden.

6. Remove the stuffed jalapenos from the oven and let them cool slightly before serving.

7. Serve the quinoa and black bean stuffed jalapenos as a spicy and satisfying appetizer or snack.

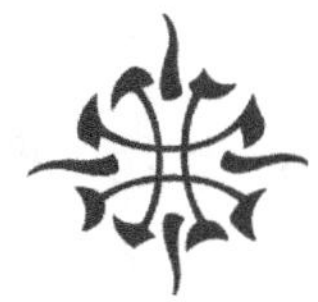

Chapter 5

Desserts

Chia Seed Pudding with Mixed Berries

Prep time: 5 minutes (plus chilling time)

Serves: 2

Ingredients:

- 1/4 cup chia seeds

- 1 cup almond milk (or any other milk of your choice)

- 1 tablespoon maple syrup (or sweetener of your choice)

- 1/2 teaspoon vanilla extract

- Mixed berries for topping (such as strawberries, blueberries, raspberries)

Directions:

1. In a bowl, combine the chia seeds, almond milk, maple syrup, and vanilla extract. Stir well to combine.

2. Cover the bowl and refrigerate for at least 2 hours or overnight, until the chia seeds have absorbed the liquid and the mixture has thickened into a pudding-like consistency.

3. Give the chia seed pudding a good stir before serving to make sure it's evenly mixed.

4. Divide the chia seed pudding into serving bowls or glasses.

5. Top with mixed berries and serve chilled. Enjoy this nutritious and delicious dessert!

Banana Nice Cream with Almond Butter

Prep time: 5 minutes

Serves: 2

Ingredients:

- 2 ripe bananas, peeled and frozen

- 2 tablespoons almond butter

- Optional toppings: chopped nuts, chocolate chips, shredded coconut

Directions:

1. Place the frozen bananas and almond butter in a blender or food processor.

2. Blend until the mixture becomes creamy and smooth, resembling the texture of soft-serve ice cream.

3. If the mixture is too thick, you can add a splash of almond milk to help with blending.

4. Once the desired consistency is reached, transfer the banana nice cream to serving bowls.

5. Top with your favorite toppings, such as chopped nuts, chocolate chips, or shredded coconut.

6. Serve immediately and enjoy this healthy and satisfying frozen treat.

DARK CHOCOLATE AVOCADO MOUSSE

Prep time: 10 minutes

Chilling time: 2 hours

Serves: 4

Ingredients:

- 2 ripe avocados

- 1/4 cup unsweetened cocoa powder

- 1/4 cup maple syrup (or sweetener of your choice)

- 1/4 cup almond milk (or any other milk of your choice)

- 1 teaspoon vanilla extract

- Optional toppings: whipped cream, berries, grated chocolate

Directions:

1. Cut the avocados in half, remove the pits, and scoop the flesh into a blender or food processor.

2. Add the cocoa powder, maple syrup, almond milk, and vanilla extract to the blender.

3. Blend until the mixture is smooth and creamy, scraping down the sides of the blender as needed.

4. Taste the mousse and adjust the sweetness if desired by adding more maple syrup.

5. Transfer the dark chocolate avocado mousse to serving dishes or glasses.

6. Cover and refrigerate for at least 2 hours to allow the mousse to set.

7. Just before serving, add your choice of toppings, such as a dollop of whipped cream, fresh berries, or grated chocolate.

8. Enjoy this rich and indulgent dessert that's packed with healthy fats from avocados.

Baked Apples with Cinnamon and Walnuts

Prep time: 10 minutes

Cooking time: 30 minutes

Serves: 4

Ingredients:

- 4 apples (such as Granny Smith or Honeycrisp)

- 2 tablespoons melted coconut oil or butter

- 2 tablespoons maple syrup (or sweetener of your choice)

- 1 teaspoon ground cinnamon

- 1/4 cup chopped walnuts

Directions:

1. Preheat the oven to 375°F (190°C). Grease a baking dish with coconut oil or butter.

2. Core the apples using an apple corer or a small knife, leaving the bottoms intact.

3. Place the cored apples in the prepared baking dish.

4. In a small bowl, combine the melted coconut oil or butter, maple syrup, and ground cinnamon.

5. Drizzle the cinnamon mixture over the apples, making sure to fill the hollowed-out centers.

6. Sprinkle the chopped walnuts over the top of the apples.

7. Bake in the preheated oven for about 25-30 minutes, or until the apples are tender and the filling is bubbly.

8. Remove from the oven and let the baked apples cool slightly before serving.

9. Serve the baked apples as is or with a scoop of vanilla ice cream for a comforting and delicious dessert.

Berry Crisp with Oat Topping

Prep time: 15 minutes

Cooking time: 30 minutes

Serves: 6

Ingredients:

For the fruit filling:

- 4 cups mixed berries (such as strawberries, blueberries, raspberries)

- 2 tablespoons maple syrup (or sweetener of your choice)

- 1 tablespoon cornstarch (or arrowroot powder)

For the oattopping:

- 1 cup rolled oats

- 1/2 cup almond flour (or regular flour)

- 1/4 cup coconut sugar (or brown sugar)

- 1/4 cup melted coconut oil or butter

- 1/2 teaspoon ground cinnamon

- Pinch of salt

Directions:

1. Preheat the oven to 350°F (175°C). Grease a baking dish with coconut oil or butter.

2. In a large bowl, combine the mixed berries, maple syrup, and cornstarch. Toss until the berries are coated evenly.

3. Transfer the berry mixture to the prepared baking dish, spreading it out evenly.

4. In another bowl, combine the rolled oats, almond flour, coconut sugar, melted coconut oil or butter, ground cinnamon, and salt. Mix until well combined and crumbly.

5. Sprinkle the oat topping evenly over the berry mixture.

6. Bake in the preheated oven for about 25-30 minutes, or until the fruit filling is bubbly and the topping is golden brown.

7. Remove from the oven and let it cool for a few minutes before serving.

8. Serve the berry crisp warm, either on its own or with a scoop of vanilla ice cream for a delightful dessert.

Vegan Chocolate Chip Cookies

Prep time: 15 minutes

Cooking time: 12 minutes

Makes: 18-20 cookies

Ingredients:

- 1/2 cup coconut oil, melted

- 3/4 cup coconut sugar (or brown sugar)

- 1/4 cup maple syrup (or agave syrup)

- 1 teaspoon vanilla extract

- 2 cups all-purpose flour

- 1/2 teaspoon baking soda

- 1/2 teaspoon salt

- 1/2 cup dairy-free chocolate chips

Directions:

1. Preheat the oven to 350°F (175°C) and line a baking sheet with parchment paper.

2. In a large mixing bowl, combine the melted coconut oil, coconut sugar, maple syrup, and vanilla extract. Stir until well combined.

3. In a separate bowl, whisk together the all-purpose flour, baking soda, and salt.

4. Add the dry ingredients to the wet ingredients and mix until a dough forms.

5. Fold in the dairy-free chocolate chips until evenly distributed throughout the dough.

6. Scoop tablespoon-sized portions of dough and roll them into balls. Place the dough balls onto the prepared baking sheet, leaving some space in between for spreading.

7. Flatten each dough ball slightly with the palm of your hand or the back of a spoon.

8. Bake in the preheated oven for about 10-12 minutes, or until the edges are golden brown.

9. Remove from the oven and let the cookies cool on the baking sheet for a few minutes before transferring them to a wire rack to cool completely.

10. Enjoy these vegan chocolate chip cookies with a glass of plant-based milk or on their own for a sweet and satisfying treat.

These desserts are all delicious and offer a variety of flavors and textures to satisfy your sweet tooth. Enjoy trying them out!

Coconut Mango Sorbet

Prep time: 10 minutes (plus freezing time)

Serves: 4

Ingredients:

- 2 ripe mangoes, peeled and chopped

- 1 can (14 ounces) full-fat coconut milk

- 1/4 cup maple syrup (or sweetener of your choice)

- 1 tablespoon lime juice

- Pinch of salt

Directions:

1. Place the chopped mangoes, coconut milk, maple syrup, lime juice, and salt in a blender or food processor.

2. Blend until the mixture is smooth and creamy.

3. Taste and adjust the sweetness or acidity by adding more maple syrup or lime juice if desired.

4. Pour the sorbet mixture into a shallow container or an ice cream maker if you have one.

5. If using a container, cover it and place it in the freezer for at least 4 hours or until the sorbet is firm.

6. If using an ice cream maker, follow the manufacturer's instructions to churn the sorbet until it reaches the desired consistency.

7. Once the sorbet is ready, scoop it into serving bowls or cones.

8. Garnish with fresh mango slices or shredded coconut if desired.

9. Enjoy this refreshing and tropical treat on a hot day!

ALMOND FLOUR BROWNIES

Prep time: 10 minutes

Cooking time: 25-30 minutes

Makes: 16 brownies

Ingredients:

- 1 cup almond flour

- 1/4 cup cocoa powder

- 1/2 teaspoon baking powder

- 1/4 teaspoon salt

- 1/2 cup coconut oil, melted

- 3/4 cup coconut sugar (or brown sugar)

- 2 large eggs

- 1 teaspoon vanilla extract

- 1/2 cup dairy-free chocolate chips (optional)

Directions:

1. Preheat the oven to 350°F (175°C) and line a square baking pan with parchment paper.

2. In a bowl, whisk together the almond flour, cocoa powder, baking powder, and salt until well combined.

3. In a separate bowl, mix together the melted coconut oil, coconut sugar, eggs, and vanilla extract until smooth.

4. Add the dry ingredients to the wet ingredients and stir until just combined.

5. If desired, fold in the chocolate chips.

6. Pour the brownie batter into the prepared baking pan and spread it out evenly.

7. Bake in the preheated oven for 25-30 minutes, or until a toothpick inserted into the center comes out with a few moist crumbs.

8. Remove from the oven and let the brownies cool completely in the pan before cutting into squares.

9. Enjoy these fudgy and decadent almond flour brownies as a healthier alternative to traditional brownies.

Lemon Poppy Seed Muffins

Prep time: 15 minutes

Cooking time: 18-20 minutes

Makes: 12 muffins

Ingredients:

- 2 cups all-purpose flour

- 1/2 cup granulated sugar

- 2 tablespoons poppy seeds

- 2 teaspoons baking powder

- 1/2 teaspoon baking soda

- 1/4 teaspoon salt

- Zest of 2 lemons

- 1 cup unsweetened almond milk (or any other milk of your choice)

- 1/2 cup freshly squeezed lemon juice

- 1/3 cup melted coconut oil or vegetable oil

- 1 teaspoon vanilla extract

Directions:

1. Preheat the oven to 375°F (190°C) and line a muffin pan with paper liners.

2. In a large bowl, whisk together the flour, sugar, poppy seeds, baking powder, baking soda, salt, and lemon zest.

3. In a separate bowl, whisk together the almond milk, lemon juice, melted coconut oil or vegetable oil, and vanilla extract.

4. Pour the wet ingredients into the dry ingredients and stir until just combined. Be careful not to overmix.

5. Divide the batter evenly among the prepared muffin cups, filling each about 2/3 full.

6. Bake in the preheated oven for 18-20 minutes, or until a toothpick inserted into the center comes out clean.

7. Remove from the oven and let the muffins cool in the pan for a few minutes before transferring them to a wire rack to cool completely.

8. These lemon poppy seed muffins are perfect for breakfast or as a light and citrusy snack.

Raspberry Coconut Chia Popsicles

Prep time: 10 minutes (plus freezing time)

Serves: 6

Ingredients:

- 1 cup fresh or frozen raspberries

- 1 can (14 ounces) full-fat coconut milk

- 2 tablespoons maple syrup (or sweetener of your choice)

- 2 tablespoons chia seeds

Directions:

1. In a blender or food processor, puree the raspberries until smooth.

2.In a bowl, combine the raspberry puree, coconut milk, maple syrup, and chia seeds. Stir well to combine.

3. Pour the mixture into popsicle molds, leaving a little bit of space at the top for expansion.

4. Place the popsicle molds in the freezer and freeze for at least 4 hours or until completely firm.

5. Once the popsicles are frozen, remove them from the molds by running the molds under warm water for a few seconds.

6. Serve immediately and enjoy these refreshing and healthy raspberry coconut chia popsicles!

Pumpkin Spice Energy Balls

Prep time: 15 minutes

Makes: 12 energy balls

Ingredients:

- 1 cup rolled oats

- 1/2 cup pumpkin puree

- 1/4 cup almond butter

- 1/4 cup honey or maple syrup

- 1/4 cup shredded coconut

- 1/4 cup chopped nuts (such as walnuts or pecans)

- 1 teaspoon pumpkin spice

- Pinch of salt

Directions:

1. In a large bowl, combine the rolled oats, pumpkin puree, almond butter, honey or maple syrup, shredded coconut, chopped nuts, pumpkin spice, and salt.

2. Stir well until all the ingredients are thoroughly combined.

3. Place the bowl in the refrigerator for about 30 minutes to allow the mixture to firm up.

4. Once the mixture has chilled, remove it from the refrigerator. Using your hands, roll the mixture into small balls, about 1 inch in diameter.

5. Place the energy balls on a baking sheet lined with parchment paper.

6. If desired, you can roll the energy balls in additional shredded coconut or pumpkin spice for added flavor.

7. Place the energy balls in an airtight container and store them in the refrigerator for up to 1 week.

8. These pumpkin spice energy balls are a delicious and nutritious snack to help boost your energy throughout the day.

GREEK YOGURT BARK WITH BERRIES AND PISTACHIOS

Prep time: 10 minutes (plus freezing time)

Serves: 4-6

Ingredients:

- 2 cups Greek yogurt

- 2 tablespoons honey or maple syrup

- 1 cup mixed berries (such as strawberries, blueberries, and raspberries)

- 1/4 cup chopped pistachios

- Optional toppings: shredded coconut, chocolate chips, or granola

Directions:

1. In a bowl, mix together the Greek yogurt and honey or maple syrup until well combined.

2. Line a baking sheet with parchment paper.

3. Pour the Greek yogurt mixture onto the lined baking sheet and spread it out evenly with a spatula.

4. Sprinkle the mixed berries and chopped pistachios over the Greek yogurt.

5. If desired, sprinkle additional toppings such as shredded coconut, chocolate chips, or granola.

6. Place the baking sheet in the freezer and freeze for at least 2-3 hours, or until the yogurt bark is completely frozen.

7. Once frozen, remove the bark from the freezer and break it into smaller pieces.

8. Serve immediately or store the Greek yogurt bark in an airtight container in the freezer for up to 1 month.

9. Enjoy this refreshing and nutritious Greek yogurt bark as a healthy dessert or snack.

Quinoa Chocolate Cake

Prep time: 15 minutes

Cooking time: 30-35 minutes

Serves: 8-10

Ingredients:

- 1 cup cooked quinoa

- 1/2 cup unsweetened cocoa powder

- 1/2 cup almond flour

- 1/2 teaspoon baking powder

- 1/2 teaspoon baking soda

- 1/4 teaspoon salt

- 3 large eggs

- 1/2 cup maple syrup or honey

- 1/4 cup melted coconut oil or vegetable oil

- 1 teaspoon vanilla extract

Directions:

1. Preheat the oven to 350°F (175°C) and grease a round cake pan.

2. In a blender or food processor, combine the cooked quinoa, cocoa powder, almond flour, baking powder, baking soda, and salt. Blend until smooth.

3. In a large bowl, whisk together the eggs, maple syrup or honey, melted coconut oil or vegetable oil, and vanilla extract.

4. Add the quinoa mixture to the wet ingredients and stir until well combined.

5. Pour the batter into the prepared cake pan and smooth the top with a spatula.

6. Bake in the preheated oven for 30-35 minutes, or until a toothpick inserted into the center comes out clean.

7. Remove the cake from the oven and let it cool in the pan for about 10 minutes before transferring it to a wire rack to cool completely.

8. Once the cake has cooled, you can frost it with your favorite frosting or serve it as is.

9. This quinoa chocolate cake is a delicious and gluten-free option for chocolate lovers

STRAWBERRY BANANA SMOOTHIE BOWL

Prep time: 5 minutes

Serves: 1

Ingredients:

- 1 frozen banana

- 1 cup frozen strawberries

- 1/2 cup almond milk (or any other milk of your choice)

- Toppings of your choice (such as sliced fresh strawberries, banana slices, granola, chia seeds, coconut flakes, or nuts)

Directions:

1. In a blender, combine the frozen banana, frozen strawberries, and almond milk.

2. Blend until smooth and creamy. If needed, add more almond milk to achieve your desired consistency.

3. Pour the smoothie into a bowl.

4. Top with your favorite toppings, such as sliced fresh strawberries, banana slices, granola, chia seeds, coconut flakes, or nuts.

5. Enjoy this refreshing and nutritious strawberry banana smoothie bowl for breakfast or as a snack.

Matcha Green Tea Ice Cream

Prep time: 10 minutes (plus freezing time)

Serves: 4

Ingredients:

- 2 cups full-fat coconut milk

- 3 tablespoons matcha green tea powder

- 1/3 cup maple syrup or honey

- 1 teaspoon vanilla extract

Directions:

1. In a blender, combine the coconut milk, matcha green tea powder, maple syrup or honey, and vanilla extract.

2. Blend until the mixture is well combined and smooth.

3. Pour the mixture into an ice cream maker and churn according to the manufacturer's instructions until it reaches a soft-serve consistency.

4. If you don't have an ice cream maker, you can pour the mixture into a shallow container and place it in the freezer.

5. Every 30 minutes, remove the container from the freezer and stir the mixture vigorously with a fork to break up any ice crystals. Repeat this process 3-4 times until the ice cream is smooth and creamy.

6. Once the ice cream reaches your desired consistency, transfer it to a lidded container and freeze for at least 4 hours or until firm.

7. Serve the matcha green tea ice cream in bowls or cones and enjoy this unique and flavorful treat.

BLUEBERRY ALMOND CRUMBLE BARS

Prep time: 15 minutes

Cooking time: 30-35 minutes

Makes: 12 bars

Ingredients:

- 2 cups rolled oats

- 1 cup almond flour

- 1/2 cup coconut oil, melted

- 1/4 cup maple syrup or honey

- 1 teaspoon vanilla extract

- 1/4 teaspoon salt

- 1 cup blueberry jam or fresh blueberries

- 1/4 cup sliced almonds

Directions:

1. Preheat the oven to 350°F (175°C) and line a square baking pan with parchment paper.

2. In a bowl, combine the rolled oats, almond flour, melted coconut oil, maple syrup or honey, vanilla extract, and salt. Mix until well combined.

3. Press two-thirds of the mixture into the bottom of the prepared baking pan to form the crust.

4. Spread the blueberry jam or scatter the fresh blueberries evenly over the crust.

5. Sprinkle the remaining oat mixture and sliced almonds over the blueberry layer.

6. Bake in the preheated oven for 30-35 minutes, or until the top is golden brown.

7. Remove from the oven and let the bars cool completely in the pan before cutting into squares.

8. These blueberry almond crumble bars are a delicious and wholesome snack or dessert option.

 Carrot Cake Bites with Cream Cheese Frosting

Prep time: 15 minutes

Makes: 12 bites

Ingredients:

For the carrot cake bites:

- 1 cup grated carrots

- 1/2 cup dates, pitted

- 1/2 cup walnuts

- 1/4 cup shredded coconut

- 1/2 teaspoon ground cinnamon

- 1/4 teaspoon ground nutmeg

- Pinch of salt

For the cream cheese frosting:

- 1/2 cup cashews, soaked for 2-3 hours and drained

- 2 tablespoons coconut cream

- 2 tablespoons maple syrup or honey

- 1 tablespoon lemon juice

- 1/2 teaspoon vanilla extract

- Pinch of salt

Directions:

1. In a food processor, combine the grated carrots, dates, walnuts, shredded coconut, ground cinnamon, ground nutmeg, and salt. Process until the mixture comes together and sticks when pressed between your fingers.

2. Roll the carrot cake mixture into bite-sized balls and place them on a plate or baking sheet lined with parchment paper. Place the bites in the refrigerator while you prepare the cream cheese frosting.

3. In a blender or food processor, combine the soaked cashews, coconut cream, maple syrup or honey, lemon juice, vanilla extract, and salt. Blend until smooth and creamy.

4. Remove the carrot cake bites from the refrigerator and drizzle the cream cheese frosting over the top of each bite.

5. Return the carrot cake bites to the refrigerator for about 30 minutes to allow the frosting to set.

6. Serve chilled and enjoy these delectable carrot cake bites with cream cheese frosting as a sweet and satisfying treat.

PEANUT BUTTER BANANA OAT BARS

Prep time: 10 minutes

Cooking time: 20-25 minutes

Makes: 12 bars

Ingredients:

- 2 cups rolled oats

- 2 ripe bananas, mashed

- 1/2 cup peanut butter

- 1/4 cup maple syrup or honey

- 1 teaspoon vanilla extract

- 1/2 teaspoon cinnamon

- 1/4 teaspoon salt

- 1/2 cup chocolate chips (optional)

Directions:

1. Preheat the oven to 350°F (175°C) and line a square baking pan with parchment paper.

2. In a large bowl, combine the rolled oats, mashed bananas, peanut butter, maple syrup or honey, vanilla extract, cinnamon, and salt. Mix until all the ingredients are well incorporated.

3. If desired, fold in the chocolate chips.

4. Press the mixture evenly into the prepared baking pan.

5. Bake in the preheated oven for 20-25 minutes or until the bars are golden brown around the edges.

6. Remove from the oven and let the bars cool completely in the pan before cutting into squares.

7. These peanut butter banana oat bars make a delicious and nutritious snack or breakfast on the go.

Chocolate Covered Strawberries

Prep time: 15 minutes

Chilling time: 30 minutes

Serves: 4

Ingredients:

- 1 pint fresh strawberries

- 6 ounces dark or semi-sweet chocolate, chopped

- Optional toppings: crushed nuts, shredded coconut, or sprinkles

Directions:

1. Rinse the strawberries and pat them dry with a paper towel. Make sure they are completely dry before dipping them in chocolate to prevent the chocolate from seizing.

2. Line a baking sheet with parchment paper.

3. Fill a small saucepan with a couple of inches of water and bring it to a simmer. Place a heatproof bowl on top of the saucepan, making sure the bottom of the bowl doesn't touch the water.

4. Add the chopped chocolate to the bowl and stir occasionally until it melts and becomes smooth.

5. Remove the bowl from the heat and let the chocolate cool for a few minutes.

6. Holding each strawberry by the stem or using a toothpick, dip it into the melted chocolate, swirling it around to coat it evenly.

7. Allow any excess chocolate to drip off, then place the chocolate-covered strawberry on the prepared baking sheet.

8. If desired, sprinkle the chocolate-covered strawberries with crushed nuts, shredded coconut, or sprinkles while the chocolate is still wet.

9. Repeat the dipping process until all the strawberries are coated in chocolate.

10. Place the baking sheet in the refrigerator for about 30 minutes, or until the chocolate has hardened.

11. Once the chocolate is firm, remove the strawberries from the refrigerator and serve.

12. Enjoy these indulgent chocolate-covered strawberries as a sweet and elegant treat.

Vanilla Bean Coconut Milk Pudding

Prep time: 5 minutes

Cooking time: 10 minutes

Chilling time: 2 hours

Serves: 4

Ingredients:

- 2 cups coconut milk

- 1/4 cup sugar

- 2 tablespoons cornstarch

- 1 vanilla bean, split and seeds scraped (or 1 teaspoon vanilla extract)

- Pinch of salt

Directions:

1. In a saucepan, combine the coconut milk, sugar, cornstarch, vanilla bean seeds (or vanilla extract), and salt. Whisk until the mixture is smooth and well combined.

2. Place the saucepan over medium heat and cook, stirring constantly, until the mixture thickens and comes to a gentle boil.

3. Reduce the heat to low and continue to cook for another 2-3 minutes, stirring constantly, until the pudding has a thick and creamy consistency.

4. Remove the saucepan from the heat and discard the vanilla bean pod, if using.

5. Pour the pudding into serving bowls or ramekins.

6. Let the pudding cool to room temperature, then cover and refrigerate for at least 2 hours, or until chilled and set.

7. Serve the vanilla bean coconut milk pudding chilled, and you can garnish it with fresh fruit, toasted coconut flakes, or a sprinkle of cinnamon if desired.

Enjoy these delightful and delicious dessert options!

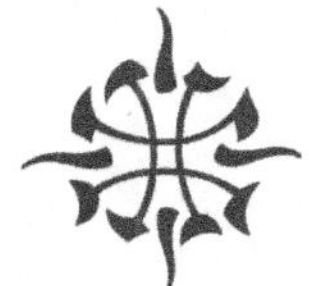

Chapter 6

Conclusion

In conclusion, this collection of dessert recipes offers a diverse range of flavors and textures to satisfy various cravings. From the refreshing Strawberry Banana Smoothie Bowl to the indulgent Chocolate Covered Strawberries, there is something for everyone. Whether you prefer fruity, creamy, or crunchy desserts, these recipes provide delicious options to enjoy. Whether you're hosting a gathering or simply treating yourself, these desserts are sure to impress. So go ahead and explore these recipes, unleash your creativity in the kitchen, and indulge in the joy of homemade desserts. Enjoy!